Dialogue About the Workforce for Population Health Improvement

PROCEEDINGS OF A WORKSHOP

Melissa Maitin-Shepard and Carla Alvarado, *Rapporteurs*

Roundtable on Population Health Improvement

Board on Population Health and Public Health Practice

Health and Medicine Division

The National Academies of
SCIENCES · ENGINEERING · MEDICINE

THE NATIONAL ACADEMIES PRESS
Washington, DC
www.nap.edu

THE NATIONAL ACADEMIES PRESS   500 Fifth Street, NW   Washington, DC 20001

This activity was supported by contracts between the National Academy of Sciences and the Association of American Medical Colleges, Blue Cross Blue Shield, The California Endowment, Dartmouth-Hitchcock Medical Center, Department of Health and Human Services' Program Support Center, Geisinger, Kaiser Permanente, The Kresge Foundation, Nemours, The Rippel Foundation, Robert Wood Johnson Foundation, Samueli Foundation, and Wake Forest Baptist Medical Center. Any opinions, findings, conclusions, or recommendations expressed in this publication do not necessarily reflect the views of any organization or agency that provided support for the project.

International Standard Book Number-13: 978-0-309-49652-0
International Standard Book Number-10: 0-309-49652-7
Digital Object Identifier: https://doi.org/10.17226/25545

Additional copies of this publication are available from the National Academies Press, 500 Fifth Street, NW, Keck 360, Washington, DC 20001; (800) 624-6242 or (202) 334-3313; http://www.nap.edu.

Copyright 2021 by the National Academy of Sciences. All rights reserved.

Printed in the United States of America

Suggested citation: National Academies of Sciences, Engineering, and Medicine. 2021. *Dialogue about the workforce for population health improvement: Proceedings of a workshop.* Washington, DC: The National Academies Press. https://doi.org/10.17226/25545.

The National Academies of
SCIENCES · ENGINEERING · MEDICINE

The **National Academy of Sciences** was established in 1863 by an Act of Congress, signed by President Lincoln, as a private, nongovernmental institution to advise the nation on issues related to science and technology. Members are elected by their peers for outstanding contributions to research. Dr. Marcia McNutt is president.

The **National Academy of Engineering** was established in 1964 under the charter of the National Academy of Sciences to bring the practices of engineering to advising the nation. Members are elected by their peers for extraordinary contributions to engineering. Dr. John L. Anderson is president.

The **National Academy of Medicine** (formerly the Institute of Medicine) was established in 1970 under the charter of the National Academy of Sciences to advise the nation on medical and health issues. Members are elected by their peers for distinguished contributions to medicine and health. Dr. Victor J. Dzau is president.

The three Academies work together as the **National Academies of Sciences, Engineering, and Medicine** to provide independent, objective analysis and advice to the nation and conduct other activities to solve complex problems and inform public policy decisions. The National Academies also encourage education and research, recognize outstanding contributions to knowledge, and increase public understanding in matters of science, engineering, and medicine.

Learn more about the National Academies of Sciences, Engineering, and Medicine at **www.nationalacademies.org**.

The National Academies of
SCIENCES · ENGINEERING · MEDICINE

Consensus Study Reports published by the National Academies of Sciences, Engineering, and Medicine document the evidence-based consensus on the study's statement of task by an authoring committee of experts. Reports typically include findings, conclusions, and recommendations based on information gathered by the committee and the committee's deliberations. Each report has been subjected to a rigorous and independent peer-review process and it represents the position of the National Academies on the statement of task.

Proceedings published by the National Academies of Sciences, Engineering, and Medicine chronicle the presentations and discussions at a workshop, symposium, or other event convened by the National Academies. The statements and opinions contained in proceedings are those of the participants and are not endorsed by other participants, the planning committee, or the National Academies.

For information about other products and activities of the National Academies, please visit www.nationalacademies.org/about/whatwedo.

PLANNING COMMITTEE ON DIALOGUE ABOUT THE WORKFORCE FOR POPULATION HEALTH IMPROVEMENT[1]

KEVIN BARNETT, Senior Investigator, Public Health Institute, and Co-Director, California Health Workforce Alliance
NISHA BOTCHWEY, Associate Professor, School of City and Regional Planning, Georgia Institute of Technology
GARY R. GUNDERSON, Vice President, Faith Health, Wake Forest Baptist Medical Center; Professor, School of Divinity, Wake Forest University
PHYLLIS D. MEADOWS, Senior Fellow, Health Program, The Kresge Foundation
JEREMY MOSELEY, Director of Community Engagement, FaithHealth Division, Wake Forest Baptist Health
KAREN MURPHY, Executive Vice President and Chief Innovation Officer, Founding Director, The Steele Institute for Health Innovation, Geisinger
JOSHUA M. SHARFSTEIN, Associate Dean for Public Health Practice and Training, Johns Hopkins Bloomberg School of Public Health

---

[1] The National Academies of Sciences, Engineering, and Medicine's planning committees are solely responsible for organizing the workshop, identifying topics, and choosing speakers. The responsibility for this published Proceedings of a Workshop rests with the workshop rapporteurs and the institution.

ROUNDTABLE ON POPULATION HEALTH IMPROVEMENT[1]

SANNE MAGNAN (*Co-Chair*), Adjunct Assistant Professor, Division of Medicine, University of Minnesota
JOSHUA M. SHARFSTEIN (*Co-Chair*), Associate Dean for Public Health Practice and Training, Johns Hopkins Bloomberg School of Public Health
PHILIP M. ALBERTI, Senior Director, Health Equity Research and Policy, Association of American Medical Colleges
TERRY ALLAN, Health Commissioner, Cuyahoga County Board of Health
JOHN AUERBACH, Executive Director, Trust for America's Health
CATHY BAASE, Chair, Board of Directors, Michigan Health Improvement Alliance; Consultant for Health Strategy, The Dow Chemical Company
DEBBIE I. CHANG, Senior Vice President, Policy and Prevention, Nemours
KATHY GERWIG, Vice President, Employee Safety, Health and Wellness and Environmental Stewardship Officer, Kaiser Permanente
MARTHE GOLD, Senior Scholar in Residence, The New York Academy of Medicine
MARC N. GOUREVITCH, Professor and Chair, Department of Population Health, New York University Langone Health
GARTH GRAHAM, President, Aetna Foundation
GARY R. GUNDERSON, Vice President, Faith Health, Wake Forest Baptist Medical Center; Professor, School of Divinity, Wake Forest University
WAYNE JONAS, Executive Director, Integrative Health Programs, H&S Ventures
ROBERT M. KAPLAN, Professor, Center for Advanced Study in the Behavioral Sciences, Stanford University
DAVID A. KINDIG, Professor Emeritus of Population Health Sciences, Emeritus Vice Chancellor for Health Sciences, School of Medicine and Public Health, University of Wisconsin–Madison
SALLY A. KRAFT, Vice President, Population Health, Dartmouth-Hitchcock
PAULA M. LANTZ, Associate Dean for Academic Affairs and Professor of Public Policy, Gerald R. Ford School of Public Policy, University of Michigan

---

[1] The National Academies of Sciences, Engineering, and Medicine's forums and roundtables do not issue, review, or approve individual documents. The responsibility for this published Proceedings of a Workshop rests with the workshop rapporteurs and the institution.

MICHELLE LARKIN, Associate Vice President, Associate Chief of Staff, Robert Wood Johnson Foundation
THOMAS A. LaVEIST, Dean, School of Public Health and Tropical Medicine, Tulane University
JEFFREY LEVI, Professor, Department of Health Policy & Management, Milken Institute School of Public Health, The George Washington University
SHARRIE McINTOSH, Vice President for Programs, New York State Health Foundation
PHYLLIS D. MEADOWS, Senior Fellow, Health Program, The Kresge Foundation
BOBBY MILSTEIN, Director, ReThink Health
JOSÉ T. MONTERO, Director, Office for State, Tribal, Local, and Territorial Support, Deputy Director, Centers for Disease Control and Prevention
KAREN MURPHY, Executive Vice President and Chief Innovation Officer, Founding Director, The Steele Institute for Health Innovation, Geisinger
MARY PITTMAN, President and Chief Executive Officer, Public Health Institute
RAHUL RAJKUMAR, Senior Vice President and Chief Medical Officer, BlueCross BlueShield of North Carolina
LOURDES J. RODRIGUEZ, Director, Community-Driven Initiatives at Dell Medical School; Associate Professor, Department of Population Health, The University of Texas at Austin
PAMELA RUSSO, Senior Program Officer, Robert Wood Johnson Foundation
MYLYNN TUFTE, State Health Officer, North Dakota Department of Health
HANH CAO YU, Chief Learning Officer, The California Endowment

Health and Medicine Division Staff
ALINA BACIU, Roundtable Director
CARLA ALVARADO, Program Officer (*until January 2021*)
KIMANI HAMILTON-WRAY, Senior Program Assistant (*through May 2019*)
BRITTANY DAVENPORT, Senior Program Assistant (*until December 2019*)
ROSE M. MARTINEZ, Senior Board Director, Board on Population Health and Public Health Practice

Consultant
MELISSA MAITIN-SHEPARD, Rapporteur

Reviewers

This Proceedings of a Workshop was reviewed in draft form by individuals chosen for their diverse perspectives and technical expertise. The purpose of this independent review is to provide candid and critical comments that will assist the National Academies of Sciences, Engineering, and Medicine in making each published proceedings as sound as possible and to ensure that it meets the institutional standards for quality, objectivity, evidence, and responsiveness to the charge. The review comments and draft manuscript remain confidential to protect the integrity of the process.

We thank the following individuals for their review of this proceedings:

PHILIP M. ALBERTI, Association of American Medical Colleges
LOURDES J. RODRIGUEZ, Dell Medical School, The University of Texas at Austin
KAREY M. SUTTON, Association of American Medical Colleges

Although the reviewers listed above provided many constructive comments and suggestions, they were not asked to endorse the content of the proceedings, nor did they see the final draft before its release. The review of this proceedings was overseen by **ANTONIA M. VILLARRUEL,** University of Pennsylvania School of Nursing. She was responsible for making certain that an independent examination of this proceedings was carried out in accordance with standards of the National Academies and that all review comments were carefully considered. Responsibility for the final content rests entirely with the rapporteurs and the National Academies.

Contents

1 **INTRODUCTION**   1
Workshop Objectives, 1
Context, 2
Organization of the Workshop and Proceedings, 3

2 **BUILDING A HEALTH WORKFORCE FOR THE FUTURE: LESSONS FROM A MULTI-STAKEHOLDER STATEWIDE INITIATIVE**   7
Discussion, 14

3 **PERSPECTIVES FROM PROFESSIONAL AND ACCREDITING ORGANIZATIONS**   17
Public Health Workforce Interest and Needs Survey, 17
Role of Essential Hospitals in Assessing Population Health Needs, 20
State of Public Health Education, 25
Local Public Health Workforce Considerations, 26
Physician Education and Health Equity, 27
Discussion, 29

4 **THE COMMUNITY HEALTH WORKFORCE**   33
Community Health Worker Panel, 33
Standardized, Scalable, and Effective Community Health Worker Programs to Improve Population Health, 35

Community Health Worker Workforce Development and
the Oregon Community Health Workers Association, 37
Community Health Worker Training and the Future of
the Profession, 40
Population Health Workforce Support for Disadvantaged
Areas Program, 42
Discussion, 44

5   **CROSS-SECTOR WORKFORCE: NATIONAL AND LOCAL EXAMPLES**   47
TRAIN Learning Network and Competencies for
Population Health Professionals, 47
Nontraditional Student Training Through the
Bloomberg American Health Initiative, 53
Planning and Public Health, 56
Health in All Policies in Fairfax County, Virginia, 58
Discussion, 60

6   **BREAKOUT SESSION: MOVING TOWARD A POPULATION HEALTH WORKFORCE EXERCISE**   63
Instructions, 63
Discussion, 64

7   **REFLECTIONS ON THE DAY AND CLOSING REMARKS**   67

APPENDIXES

A   References   71
B   Workshop Agenda   73
C   Biosketches of Speakers, Moderators, and Planning Committee
Members   77
D   Small Group Exercise Instructions and Worksheet   93

1

Introduction[1]

On March 21, 2019, the Roundtable on Population Health Improvement of the National Academies of Sciences, Engineering, and Medicine (the National Academies) convened a 1-day workshop to explore the broad and multi-disciplinary nature of the population health workforce. The workshop was held at the Keck Center of the National Academies in Washington, DC, and organized by a planning committee made up of members of the Roundtable on Population Health Improvement and population health experts (see Appendix B for the workshop agenda).

WORKSHOP OBJECTIVES

The main objectives of the workshop were to explore the following three topics that resulted from the Statement of Task for the workshop (see Box 1-1):

1. Facilitating a population health orientation/perspective among public health and health care leaders and professionals;

---

[1] This workshop was organized by an independent planning committee whose role was limited to identification of topics and speakers. This Proceedings of a Workshop was prepared by the rapporteurs as a factual summary of the presentations and discussions that took place at the workshop. Statements, recommendations, and opinions expressed are those of individual presenters and participants and are not necessarily endorsed or verified by the National Academies of Sciences, Engineering, and Medicine; the Health and Medicine Division; or the roundtable, and they should not be construed as reflecting any group consensus.

> **BOX 1-1**
> **Workshop Statement of Task**
>
> An ad hoc planning committee will plan and convene a 1-day public workshop that will explore the broad and multi-disciplinary nature of the population health workforce. The workshop may include presentations about (1) fomenting a population health orientation/perspective among public health and health care leaders and professionals; (2) framing the work of personnel such as community health workers, health navigators, and peer-to-peer chronic disease management educators within the context of population health; and (3) leveraging the competencies of other (nonmedical and non–public health) workforces, such as education, transportation, and planning, within the public and private sectors working to include a "health in all policies," community livability, or well-being orientation in their activities. A proceedings of the presentations and discussion at the workshop will be prepared by a designated rapporteur in accordance with institutional guidelines.

2. Framing the work of personnel such as community health workers (CHWs), health navigators, and peer-to-peer chronic disease management educators within the context of population health; and
3. Leveraging the competencies of public- and private-sector workforces, such as education, transportation, and planning, that are working to include a "health in all policies," community livability, or well-being orientation in their activities.

CONTEXT

Sanne Magnan from the University of Minnesota opened the workshop by providing background on the Roundtable for Population Health Improvement, the need for the workshop, and the workshop's goals.

She explained that since February 2013, the Roundtable on Population Health Improvement[2] has provided a trusted venue for leaders from the public and private sectors to meet and discuss leverage points and opportunities arising from changes in the social and political environment for achieving better population health. She added that the roundtable's vision is of a strong, healthy, and productive society that cultivates human capital and equal opportunity. This vision rests on the recognition that out-

---

[2] More information about the Roundtable on Population Health Improvement is available at http://nationalacademies.org/HMD/Activities/PublicHealth/PopulationHealth ImprovementRT.aspx (accessed May 10, 2021).

comes such as improved life expectancy, quality of life, and health for all are shaped by interdependent social, economic, environmental, genetic, behavioral, and health care factors and will require robust national and community-based policies and dependable resources to achieve.

The National Academies have produced reports on workforce topics relevant to improving population health, including *Transforming the Workforce for Children Birth Through Age 8: A Unifying Foundation* (IOM and NRC, 2015) and *Communities in Action: Pathways to Health Equity* (NASEM, 2017). Magnan explained that rather than focusing on workforce development, the workshop explored broad strategies for helping many kinds of current and future workers understand how they can directly or indirectly contribute to population health and well-being.

Magnan referred to the spectrum of opportunities and strategies for introducing, communicating, sharing, and teaching population health knowledge—ranging from basic, practical concepts to specialized graduate school curricula—that are already available to a wide range of practitioners, students, and audiences (see Figure 1-1). The workshop sought to address three broad categories of the workforce for population health: (1) the traditional health sector workforce in public health and health care settings; (2) the community workforce, such as community health navigators and CHWs; and (3) the workforce in other sectors, such as education, planning, and business. Magnan pointed out that some of these workers may consider themselves population health workers, while others may not.

Magnan noted that the National Academies were conducting two consensus studies that include the discussion of workforce dimensions: *Integrating Social Care into the Delivery of Health Care: Moving Upstream to Improve the Nation's Health* (NASEM, 2019a) and *Vibrant and Healthy Kids: Aligning Science, Practice, and Policy to Advance Health Equity* (NASEM, 2019b). Magnan concluded by stating that the work of the roundtable "magnifies and reinforces that the workforce for population health presents in many formal and informal ways" and that the workshop objectives emphasize the broad thinking needed for the future workforce.

ORGANIZATION OF THE WORKSHOP AND PROCEEDINGS

This proceedings summarizes the presentations and discussions that took place during the public workshop. The first presentation was a keynote address focused on lessons from a multi-stakeholder statewide initiative for building a health workforce for the future. The keynote was followed by three panels, each addressing one of the workshop objectives. The panels included a mix of presentations, discussion, and question-and-answer sessions with members of the audience. A small group exercise in the latter part of the workshop provided an opportunity for workshop

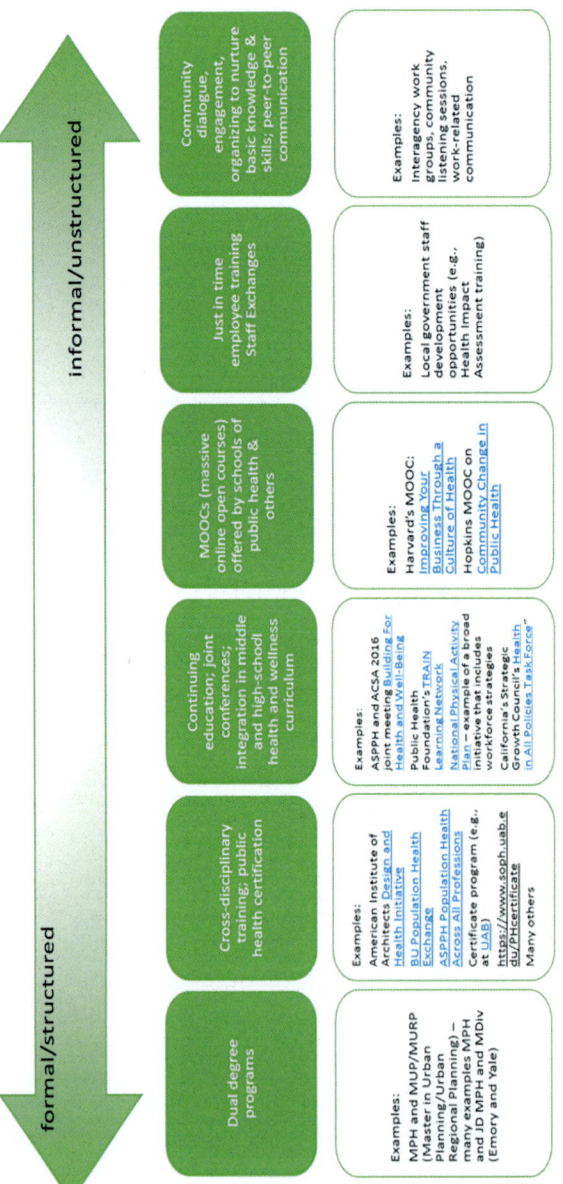

FIGURE 1-1 Toward a population health workforce.
NOTES: The term "population health workforce" does not refer to creating the workforce de novo. It is about helping many kids of workers and future workers understand how they can and do contribute to population health and well-being either directly or indirectly. This figure illustrates the spectrum of opportunities and model strategies for introducing, communicating, sharing, and teaching population health knowledge—ranging from basic practical concepts to specialized graduate school curricula—to a wide range of practitioners, students, and audiences. This is for illustration only and is not intended to be comprehensive. Also, others may choose to name or order the categories differently, to classify activities differently, or provide different examples. ACSA = Associate of Collegiate Schools of Architecture; ASPPH = Association of Schools and Programs of Public Health; BU = Boston University; JD = Juris Doctor; MDiv = Master of Divinity; MOOC = massive open online course; MPH = Master in Public Health; MUP = Master in Urban Planning; MURP = Master in Urban Regional Planning; NAS = National Academy of Sciences; UAB = The University of Alabama at Birmingham.
SOURCE: Magnan presentation, March 22, 2019.

participants to consider how they could use population health workforce strategies to respond to the health-related problems of school absenteeism, lack of affordable housing, and food insecurity in communities. The workshop concluded with reflections from roundtable members and participants on key takeaways from the day's presentations and discussions.

2

Building a Health Workforce for the Future: Lessons from a Multi-Stakeholder Statewide Initiative[1]

Kevin Barnett from the Public Health Institute and the California Health Workforce Alliance delivered the keynote address. Barnett opened by explaining that he began working on the issue of health workforce diversity in California 16 years ago and had previously participated in an Institute of Medicine committee led by Brian Smedley that produced a report on increasing the diversity of the health professions (IOM, 2004). That study explored the topic of holding health profession educational institutions responsible for building a diverse health workforce in the future.

Following that process, Barnett and his colleague Jeff Oxendine launched an initiative called Connecting the Dots, which had the goal of developing a comprehensive strategy to build the health workforce of the future. The project was supported by The California Endowment and was completed in 2008. Since then, Barnett and colleagues have convened diverse stakeholders across California, including employers, academic institutions, and advocates, to identify ways to advance the strategy.

Barnett recounted that in 2017, he and Oxendine were approached by the five largest foundations in California, which asked if they were interested in creating a comprehensive health workforce master plan, which he had recommended be developed back in 2005. The five foundation funders included the Blue Shield of California Foundation, The California

---

[1] This section summarizes information presented by Kevin Barnett from the Public Health Institute and the California Health Workforce Alliance. The statements made are not endorsed or verified by the National Academies of Sciences, Engineering, and Medicine.

Endowment, the California Health Care Foundation, The California Wellness Foundation, and the Gordon and Betty Moore Foundation. He noted it was significant that the five foundations that supported the work have slightly different priorities and emphasis, but they came together to support a common goal—an exemplary type of philanthropic collaboration.

Barnett's presentation described the process used to develop this plan, beginning with the foundational questions that were addressed as part of the project:

- What are key gaps in the health workforce pathway?
- What is a vision to meet workforce needs that will improve population health?
- Why is health workforce diversity essential to improving population health?
- How are other sectors crucial to improving population health?
- What is a holistic way to approach health workforce development?
- Who has a role in building the health workforce of the future?

The questions yielded the charge of the newly formed commission, which included developing a strategic plan, creating implementation strategies, leveraging existing efforts, and engaging stakeholders (see Box 2-1).

Barnett pointed out it was important for the commission to think both in the short term about providing access to clinical health care services, and in the long term about addressing the real drivers of poor health. The

---

BOX 2-1
Charge of the California Future Health Workforce Commission

Presented by Kevin Barnett

- Develop a strategic plan to build the future California health workforce (2030).
  - Advance practical short-, medium-, and long-term solutions to address current and future workforce gaps.
  - Agree on a cooperative strategy that promotes shared ownership and priorities and that makes optimal use of diverse stakeholder resources.
- Secure commitments for effective plan implementation, including a state infrastructure to facilitate and monitor progress.
- Build on, align with, and leverage relevant public and private efforts for greater collective innovation, efficiency, and impact.
- Educate and engage key public and private stakeholders to support success.

commission had to consider legislative and executive branch solutions and ways that all sectors could come together to address the issue. The commission also had to secure commitments for effective plan implementation that went beyond simply developing a report or list of potential solutions. Key elements noted to drive the process included dialogue, rationale for data, and evidence.

The commission had three core areas of focus, which were the topics that it determined were most important and urgent: (1) primary care and prevention, (2) behavioral health, and (3) healthy aging and care for older adults. Other issues could be added later as needed. The commission was concerned with how to build a workforce of the future that reflected California's increasingly diverse communities. As Barnett explained, the overriding issues were the misdistribution of health professionals to serve rural and disadvantaged urban communities and the role of technology in driving it.

Barnett next described some of the challenges faced in California, which he sees elsewhere in the country as well. As he explained, in the next 10 years, the state is expected to have 41 percent fewer psychiatrists than needed and a shortfall of more than 4,000 primary care clinicians and up to 600,000 home care workers. He provided examples of some of the potential drivers. For example, Latinx people represent approximately 40 percent of the state's population but only 7 percent of physicians, contributing to the 7 million Californians—primarily people of color—who live in areas of health profession shortage. In addition, California's provider–population ratios, particularly in inner-city and rural areas, are only about half the federal recommended levels. Compounding the situation is that one-third of practitioners and nurse practitioners (NPs) are over age 55 and are expected to retire within 10 years. Barnett noted that these statistics are even more dire in rural areas.

Barnett also provided similar statistics regarding the public health workforce. He explained that more than 60 percent of senior leadership of public health agencies is eligible for retirement. He added that more than 95 percent of the funding for the state's public health department is categorical.

Barnett provided some statistics regarding California's aging population to illustrate the extent of the problem and the importance of acting. He explained that an additional 4 million Californians will reach retirement age by 2030, almost a 90 percent increase from 2012. Barnett was particularly struck that a large percentage of these people live alone, implying that there may be additional challenges in ensuring that they receive the care they need. He added that more than half of these individuals rely on Social Security for more than 80 percent of their income.

Barnett also highlighted challenges with access to behavioral and mental health services, as emergency department visits related to mental health disorders increased by more than 50 percent nationally between 2006 and 2013.

Barnett sees similar challenges with provider training cost and capacity. Barnett explained that with 60 percent of California's medical students attending school out of state, California relies on other states to educate its physicians and on them choosing to return to California afterward. However, he noted that many do not come back due to California's high cost of living and other factors. The high cost of medical education and the higher prestige of specialties versus primary care also drive many students toward specialties. Barnett noted that California has one of the most extensive teaching health center graduate medical education training programs in the country, with six federally qualified health centers (FQHCs) providing this training. However, Barnett added, the providers that run these programs are often already stretched thin and take additional time away from clinical care to support their students.

Barnett also described challenges related to the social determinants of health. The homeless population in California has increased more than 50 percent in the past 5 years, with nearly one-quarter of the homeless population in the United States, or close to 60,000 people, living in Los Angeles alone. That has led to a 12-year waiting list for Section 8 housing and a need for an additional 1.5 million units of rental housing. He explained that close to 40 percent of the state's population lives at or below 150 percent of the California Poverty Metric, which is based on the federal poverty level but increased to account for the higher cost of living in California. Barnett also explained that while there is a commitment to providing access to preschool, the state falls short in doing so. He noted that this is important because lack of education early in life "establishes the circumstances under which it is difficult for many of these children to pursue career and health professions, as well as an income that will support them and their families."

An additional challenge is that California is 49th in the country in reimbursement under MediCal, the state's Medicaid program. Providers not tied to an FQHC provide services under MediCal at highly discounted rates. Technology is also not equitably distributed across the state. Barnett explained that the health care delivery system and its linkages do not currently have the capacity to provide and extend the reach of the provider population to address these issues in low-income communities. He commented that in the future there should be an increased investment in K–12 education.

Barnett next spoke about the California Future Health Workforce Commission's structure and processes. The 24-member commission was co-chaired by Lloyd Dean, chief executive officer of Dignity Health (now

CommonSpirit), and Janet Napolitano, president of the University of California. Most of the other commissioners were decision makers who could provide influence and command resources, including respected chancellors and presidents of higher education institutions in the state and State Senate and State Assembly health committee chairs. There was also a 40-member Technical Advisory Committee (TAC) made up of leaders and experts in the workforce arena who understood the issues and could provide insights as the process moved forward. Committee members were organized into three subcommittees, each addressing a priority area. Between September 2017 and January 2019, the commission met seven times; the TAC also met during that time.

Barnett explained that as a part of the process, the commission also conducted a statewide survey to gather input on an extensive set of draft recommendations. As of April 2018, there were 177 recommendations, which were reduced to 27. On January 15, 2019, the commission adopted the final report with its 27 recommendations (California Future Health Workforce Commission, 2019).[2] Ten of them were identified as top priorities for implementation. Barnett noted that the commission is actively engaged in promoting the public report.

Barnett next described certain elements of the commission's deliberative process. He emphasized that the commission spent a significant amount of time initially "blue sky visioning," asking questions such as "Where do we want to go? … Where do we want our institutions to be? What kinds of transformation do we want? What [is that] going to look like by 2030?" Other elements included identifying and analyzing problems, defining success and end products, establishing strategies, engaging stakeholders, analyzing and refining strategy, developing recommendations, conducting impact assessments, and selecting top recommendations.

Barnett also described some highlights of the process used to develop the recommendations (see Figure 2-1). The subcommittees conducted an initial review of information and brought key takeaways to the TAC for its input and then to the commission for refinement. He noted that the commission co-chairs played a particularly pivotal role in establishing the final priorities near the end of the process.

The commission's final recommendations included three main strategies and reflected the need for a comprehensive approach:

- Strategy 1, "increase opportunities for all Californians to pursue health careers," was focused on how to create opportunities early

---

[2] The Commission's full report, recommendations, and impact statements are available at https://futurehealthworkforce.org (accessed May 10, 2021).

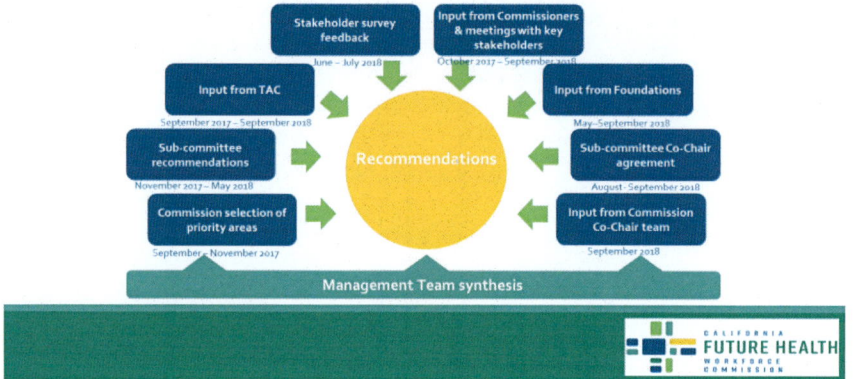

FIGURE 2-1 California Future Health Workforce Commission's process to develop recommendations.
SOURCE: Barnett presentation, March 22, 2019.

on in careers and build the health career pathways that provide opportunities to pursue higher education.
- Strategy 2, "align and expand education and training to meet Californians' needs," referred to necessary changes in the higher education process.
- Strategy 3, "strengthen the capacity, effectiveness, and retention of the health workforce," was related to building the capacity and effectiveness of the current workforce to better serve communities (see Box 2-2).

Barnett next shared the commission's recommendations for achieving each of the three main strategies, highlighting the top priorities (see Box 2-2). He emphasized the broad spectrum of recommendations and synergistic linkages between many of them. As he noted, some recommendations may be related to K–12 education and some to higher education, but all are focused on equity and addressing the underinvestment in rural and inner-city areas and underserved populations. With respect to education and training needs, Barnett noted an emphasis on drawing people from underserved communities, particularly communities of color, and supporting them in returning to and practicing in these communities after their training.

Barnett mentioned that the commission largely focused on delivery of clinical services. He explained that because there had been pent-up demand over several years to address access to primary and behavioral health care, those issues took precedence and were prioritized. However, he pointed out that scaling engagement of community health workers

> **BOX 2-2**
> **Strategies Proposed by the California Future Health Workforce Commission**
>
> **Presented by Kevin Barnett**
>
> **Strategy 1: Increase Opportunities for All Californians to Pursue Health Careers**
> 1.1 Scale pipeline programs for students from underrepresented and low-income backgrounds.
> 1.2 Recruit and support underrepresented college students to pursue health careers.
> 1.3 Support scholarships for priority professions and service in underserved communities.
>
> **Strategy 2: Align and Expand Education and Training to Meet Californians' Needs**
> 2.1 Sustain and expand the Programs in Medical Education program across University of California campuses.
> 2.2 Expand the number of primary care physician and psychiatry residency positions.
> 2.3 Recruit and train students from underserved communities to practice in community health centers in home regions.
>
> **Strategy 3: Strengthen the Capacity, Effectiveness, and Retention of the Health Workforce**
> 3.1 Maximize the role of nurse practitioners (NPs) to fill gaps in primary care.
> 3.2 Establish a universal home care worker family of jobs with career ladders and training.
> 3.3 Develop a psychiatric NP program that serves underserved rural and urban communities.
> 3.4 Scale the engagement of community health workers, *promotores*, and peer providers.

(CHWs) and peer providers was identified as a top priority. Subcommittees and other leaders on the issue were also convened to develop this recommendation. Barnett explained that while there is "a fairly extensive network of *promotores* and CHWs in California, for the most part, the engagement of these workers by ... mainstream providers is relatively limited; ... their roles are relatively circumscribed." Within this recommendation, Barnett pointed to "significant emphasis on understanding the comprehensive role CHWs could play not only in managing the care of individual patients but also working in and with communities to ... begin to address the drivers of poor health, including working in the areas of policy advocacy." He highlighted relevant issues, such as quality of housing and indoor environmental factors.

Barnett described a few other specific recommendations of the commission, including the recommendation to build the capacity of local public health agencies to support collaborative community health improvement. As he explained, that recommendation reflected a commitment to shared ownership and involved the state establishing a fund and making part of it available to match money provided by local hospitals and health systems. The funding could be used to engage someone with epidemiological expertise, preferably social epidemiological expertise, to connect the "parallel play" of each health care provider's community benefit programs and activities, work toward focusing and aligning these efforts in communities with inequities, and provide accountability for making progress on addressing the priority issues.

Barnett explained that the recommendations reflect the overall commitment of the commission to address changes to not only the health care system but other sectors, including the community development sector, and to establish relationships between health care and other sectors. Important steps in developing the recommendations involved budgeting, conducting impact assessments, and considering where available data may be limited.

In closing, Barnett described next steps for disseminating and beginning to implement the commission's recommendations. He noted that there would be an upcoming hearing, presentations to State Senate committees, and possible introduction of state legislation to address some of the recommendations. The five foundation funders are also considering ways to provide continued support for facilitation, monitoring, and ensuring that state infrastructure is sufficient to move the process forward. Employers and academic institutions in California are also being asked to consider their role in the process, in terms of the allocation of resources and their priorities to reflect the report recommendations.

DISCUSSION

Following Barnett's presentation, there was a brief discussion with the audience. Donna Grande from the American College of Preventive Medicine asked Barnett for his top recommendations for congressional action in the next 3–5 years. Barnett noted that one priority is increasing investment in K–12 education in low-income communities. He elaborated by stating that increasing diversity in the health workforce requires early investment in pre-K education, targeted outreach and engagement, and support of people in low-income communities. He also pointed to the maldistribution of resources in K–12 education, with people in middle-class and affluent communities providing additional support to schools in low-income communities. Barnett believes this has led public schools to become "the most segregated institutions in our communities."

Barnett noted that a second priority is moving from the "legacy model of health care delivery" to "fully integrating the social determinants of health into all ... health profession education institutions, not as a course but as an ongoing part of the education process."

Barnett suggested that an additional priority could be targeted training in communities and support systems for more providers to practice in rural and inner-city communities. He recommended substantial increases in funding for government public health and other entities that move away from categorical program silos and provide for more dynamic collaboration with a broad spectrum of stakeholders.

Sanne Magnan asked whether the committee discussed changing workforce needs related to baby boomers and the increase in lay health workers, and how to capitalize on these trends to address population health improvement. Barnett responded by explaining that the increase in home health care workers was addressed in several of the commission's recommendations. In addition, the committee recognized that many retirees are still healthy and want to support population health improvement through strategies such as working in home care or mentoring young people. Magnan also noted that she appreciated Barnett's emphasis on the diversity of the health care workforce, including not only primary care physicians but also NPs, psychiatrists, and CHWs. In response, Barnett pointed out that the commission's recommendations included a strong emphasis on NPs, and work is under way to provide NPs with full practice authority, which they have in 22 states, including California. His group also discussed physician assistants playing a critical role in the California health care workforce, but this was not addressed in the commission's report. Points made by the keynote speaker are highlighted below (see Box 2-3).

BOX 2-3
Points Made by Kevin Barnett

- An exemplary type of philanthropic collaboration is multiple funders with slightly different priorities and emphasis coming together to support a common goal.
- It was important for the California Future Health Workforce Commission to consider both short-term needs regarding access to clinical health care services and long-term needs regarding the real drivers of poor health.
- Public health and health care provider shortfalls, unaddressed social determinants of health, and an aging population all present challenges for the public health and health care workforce in California, and likely elsewhere.

NOTE: This list is the rapporteurs' summary of the main points made by the individual speaker and does not reflect any consensus among workshop participants or endorsement by the National Academies of Sciences, Engineering, and Medicine.

3

Perspectives from Professional and Accrediting Organizations[1]

The next session was the first of three panel sessions and focused on the perspectives of professional and accrediting organizations. The session was moderated by Phyllis Meadows from The Kresge Foundation and featured presentations by Brian Castrucci from the de Beaumont Foundation and Kalpana Ramiah from America's Essential Hospitals (AEH). Following these presentations, Laura Rasar King from the Council on Education for Public Health (CEPH), Kaye Bender from the Public Health Accreditation Board (PHAB), and Lisa Howley from the Association of American Medical Colleges (AAMC) served as discussants. There was also an opportunity for discussion with other workshop attendees in the audience.

PUBLIC HEALTH WORKFORCE INTEREST AND NEEDS SURVEY[2]

Brian Castrucci opened by providing a brief background on the de Beaumont Foundation, explaining that it focuses on "the people, the policies, and the partnerships that [are necessary] for communities to achieve their optimal health." His presentation addressed the governmen-

---

[1] This chapter summarizes information presented by panel session speakers. The statements made are not endorsed or verified by the National Academies of Sciences, Engineering, and Medicine.
[2] This section summarizes information presented by Brian Castrucci from the de Beaumont Foundation. The statements made are not endorsed or verified by the National Academies of Sciences, Engineering, and Medicine.

tal public health workforce, which he called "the backbone of a healthy community."

To provide context on his perspective, Castrucci explained that prior to joining the Foundation, he worked in state and local public health agencies. He noted that the Foundation would often consult state health officials when seeking to understand the needs of governmental public health agencies. However, he added, due to their limited tenure or lack of prior experience in governmental settings, these officials' answers did not fully capture the needs of the public health workforce. As Castrucci explained, this led the Foundation to create the Public Health Workforce Interests and Needs Survey (PH WINS) "to capture the ideas, thoughts, [and] challenges of the other 99.9 percent of the workforce."

The PH WINS was first conducted in 2014 in 37 states and received more than 10,000 responses. A pilot conducted among local public health agencies added approximately 10,000 more responses. In 2017, the Foundation conducted the survey with 47 state health agencies and a nationally representative sample of local health departments, and had more than 47,000 respondents. Castrucci noted that the detailed findings from the 2017 survey were published in the March 2019 supplement in the *Journal of Public Health Management and Practice* (PH WINS, 2019). His presentation at the workshop focused on key high-level findings from the 2017 survey, implications, and next steps.[3]

According to Castrucci, the survey found high levels of job satisfaction in the public health workforce. However, many workers were considering leaving their jobs in the next year. He noted that this was due to workers nearing retirement age and younger people departing their jobs. The survey also found that most workers were satisfied with their jobs but not equally satisfied with their pay. There was also a high level of worker engagement.

The survey found that the top training needs of workers at all levels in administration and management, including executives, managers, and frontline staff, were budget and finance. Castrucci provided an anecdote using his own experience as an epidemiologist earlier in his career, noting that while he was skilled in research and analysis, he did not know about benefits or budgeting. He explained that he felt well prepared to work as an epidemiologist but had not been trained to be a leader, manager, or businessperson, yet these were aspects of his job.

Castrucci next provided some statistics comparing the demographics of the public health workforce with those of the U.S. workforce as a whole. The public health workforce is primarily (79 percent) female; however, 4

---

[3] More information about the PH WINS is available at https://www.debeaumont.org/ph-wins (accessed May 10, 2021).

out of every 100 male workers reach the highest levels of leadership, versus only 2 women. The workforce is also primarily white and much older than the U.S. workforce, with 45 percent over 50 years of age and 10 percent under 30, presenting a challenge when the large number of older workers retires. Castrucci noted that the public health workforce is also well educated, with older workers more likely to have a bachelor's degree as their highest degree and younger workers more likely to have a master's degree.

As Castrucci mentioned earlier, nearly half the public health workforce (47 percent) is considering leaving an organization, an increase of 41 percent between 2014 and 2017. He elaborated that 22 percent of workers are planning to retire, noting that these are people who say they plan to retire, not simply that they have reached retirement age. Castrucci highlighted as particularly concerning the 25 percent of workers who say they plan to leave their job in the next year for reasons other than retirement.

Castrucci outlined the top five reasons that workers leave: (1) inadequate pay, (2) lack of advancement, (3) workplace environment, (4) low job satisfaction, and (5) lack of support. He noted that except for pay, all of these reasons are within management's control in a health department or organization. While public health may not be able to compete on pay with health care systems, Castrucci suggested that it could ensure there are opportunities for advancement or stretch assignments and provide a solid work environment. Castrucci highlighted the paradox that while job satisfaction is high (81 percent), satisfaction with pay is low (48 percent).

As Castrucci explained, the survey found that the public health workforce is mission driven. In the 2014 survey, 98 percent of respondents agreed with the statement that they pursued a public health career because they wanted to make a difference. This question was not asked in 2017 because there was such high agreement on the first survey. The PH WINS inquired about drivers of workforce engagement, and Castrucci noted that there were individual-level factors, such as having high motivation and believing that the work being carried out is important and related to the agency's goals and priorities.

He added that there are also management-level factors that require attention. He was particularly concerned that only 44 percent of respondents said that "creativity and innovation are rewarded" in their workplace, emphasizing that the workforce has a large number of people with master's degrees. For example, after participating in a learning collaborative that the Foundation convened, South Carolina was able to change its statistics regarding support for creativity and innovation.

Castrucci next described some ways the Foundation is addressing the problems identified in the survey. To address budget- and finance-related training needs, the Foundation has partnered with the University of Miami to create a program called Building Essentials in Administration and Management, a $500 certificate course for people working in governmental public health. Castrucci suggested that public health end its assessments of needs and gaps and focus on addressing the already identified needs and gaps.

With respect to emerging concepts in public health, Castrucci noted that only 43 percent of respondents said that multi-sector partnerships were important to their work, and only 35 percent had even heard of "health in all policies," highlighting the need for more training in these areas. Digging deeper into operationalizing both concepts, Castrucci noted that 85 percent of respondents said that their agency should be involved in health equity. However, only 63 percent thought their agency should be involved in affecting the K–12 system, 53 percent for transportation, 55 percent for the built environment, and 56 percent for the economy.

ROLE OF ESSENTIAL HOSPITALS IN ASSESSING POPULATION HEALTH NEEDS[4]

Kalpana Ramiah from the Essential Hospitals Institute at AEH opened her presentation with background on the organization.[5] She explained that AEH is an association of nearly 300 member hospitals across the country linked by their mission to serve vulnerable populations. There are four other common characteristics of AEH's member hospitals:

1. Providing comprehensive, coordinated care through primary care and specialty care networks;
2. Training, with member hospitals training more than three times as many physicians and clinicians as other U.S. hospitals;
3. Providing specialized life-saving care, such as trauma care, burn care, and neonatal intensive care unit services, with essential hospitals operating about one-third of the level one trauma centers and 40 percent of the burn care beds in large cities; and
4. Focusing on advancing public health (the organization was previously called the National Association of Public Hospitals, and many of its member hospitals still operate or function as part of public health departments).

---

[4] This section summarizes information presented by Kalpana Ramiah from AEH. The statements made are not endorsed or verified by the National Academies of Sciences, Engineering, and Medicine.

[5] More information about AEH and its resources is available at https://essentialcommunities.org (accessed May 10, 2021).

Ramiah showed a map of the United States that illustrated the prevalence of individuals with claims for three or more chronic conditions, highlighting the differences in color across the country, or the uneven distribution of chronic diseases. She then showed the same map (see Figure 3-1) with added red dots to indicate the locations of AEH member hospitals, highlighting that they are concentrated in the areas with the highest rates of patients with complex needs.

Ramiah pointed out that essential hospitals provide nine times more uncompensated care than other U.S. hospitals, which translates to a margin of 1.6 percent compared with 7.8 percent for hospitals overall. She noted that this statistic would be worse off and reach –3 percent if it were not for the disproportionate share hospital[6] payment that these hospitals receive. In addition, many patients in communities served by essential hospitals also have social needs. This includes 25.3 million individuals who are below the poverty line, 19.4 million without health insurance, 10.1 million with limited access to healthy food, and 350,000 who are homeless (Roberson and Ramiah, 2018). Social determinants of health are major issues in essential hospitals.

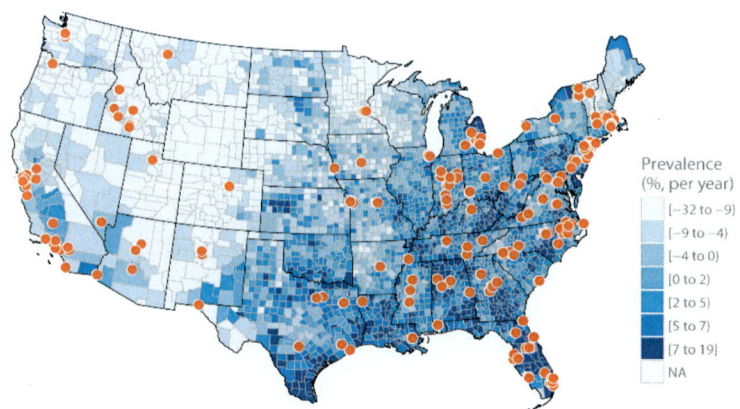

FIGURE 3-1 Prevalence of three or more claims-based conditions, 2015, and location of AEH member hospitals.
SOURCES: Ramiah presentation, March 22, 2019; CMS, 2016.

---

[6] Disproportionate share hospitals serve a significantly disproportionate number of low-income patients and receive payments from the Centers for Medicaid & Medicare Services to cover the costs of providing care to uninsured patients. See the Health Resources and Services Administration's factsheet at https://www.cms.gov/Outreach-and-Education/Medicare-Learning-Network-MLN/MLNProducts/Downloads/Disproportionate_Share_Hospital.pdf (accessed May 10, 2021).

Ramiah described a model (see Figure 3-2), adapted from a model by Hester et al. (2015) at the Centers for Disease Control and Prevention (CDC), to explain what essential hospitals do in population health. Level 1.0 is episodic nonintegrated care: the patient arrives, is treated, and leaves the hospital. Level 2.0 is the coordinated care system with outcome-accountable care, in which the hospital cares for patients and is also responsible for making sure that they continue to take their medication after they leave. Level 3.0 is community-integrated health care that goes beyond direct medical care to focus on the community. In levels 1.0 and 2.0, the hospital is only concerned with the patient population, but in level 3.0, it addresses the health of the whole community. AEH defines community-integrated health care as a strategy through which health care providers work with other sectors in both complementary and collaborative ways to promote health.

To further illustrate this concept, Ramiah showed a chart (see Figure 3-3) examining the spectrum of community-integrated care. Guiding the audience through the figure, Ramiah provided examples of the activities a member hospital might carry out and where these would be on the quadrants. For example, providing food for patients is a downstream intervention that is just for patients. As another example, opening a food bank for the community is a downstream intervention in the community because, while it is available to all community members, it does not fully address the social determinants of food access and affordability (see Figure 3-3).

Ramiah explained that AEH acknowledges that their member hospitals may have to operate in all three levels. She emphasized that her orga-

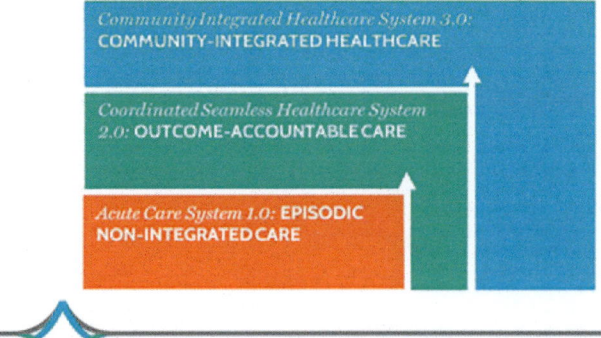

FIGURE 3-2 What is population health?
NOTE: CIHC = community integrated health care.
SOURCES: Ramiah presentation, March 22, 2019; adapted from Hester et al., 2015.

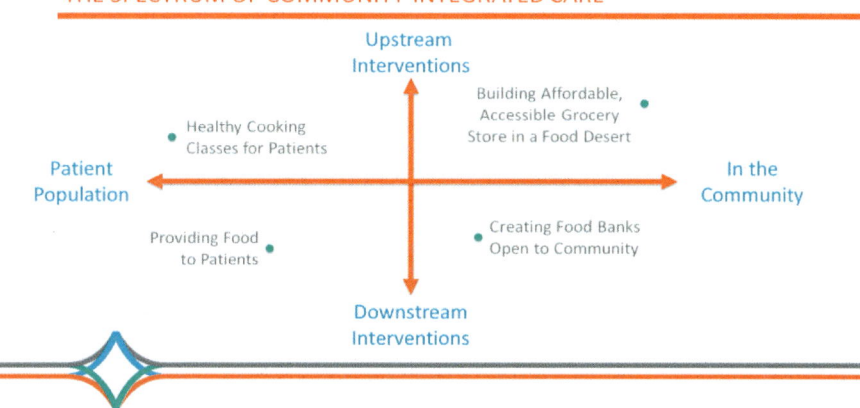

FIGURE 3-3 The spectrum of community-integrated care.
SOURCE: Ramiah presentation, March 22, 2019.

nization sees the spectrum of community-integrated care as just that—a spectrum.

Ramiah next provided information about AEH and what the organization does to support its members. It provides research, education, leadership development, and policy and advocacy. In 2015–2016, it engaged in a strategic initiative related to population health; conducted member surveys, expert interviews, and key informant interviews within its membership; and held a deliberative summit to understand what member hospitals are doing in population health, what they mean by population health, and facilitators and barriers in this work.

Ramiah provided some highlights from the research (AEH, 2016). AEH received survey responses from 106 hospitals and conducted interviews to obtain additional information (see Figure 3-4). In response to questions about additional resources needed for population health improvement activities, the top request was additional funding, particularly funding that was sustainable and not grant dependent. The second most requested resources were data and analytical tools that facilitated data sharing. The next three resource requests related to human capital, including staff training, leadership, and additional staff.

Ramiah next described work funded by The Kresge Foundation examining job descriptions of population health executives in AEH member hospitals, such as directors and vice presidents. AEH conducted interviews and focus groups with them. Ramiah was surprised to learn that many of them did not have job descriptions and that population health was a "one-person department" at a number of hospitals. In addition,

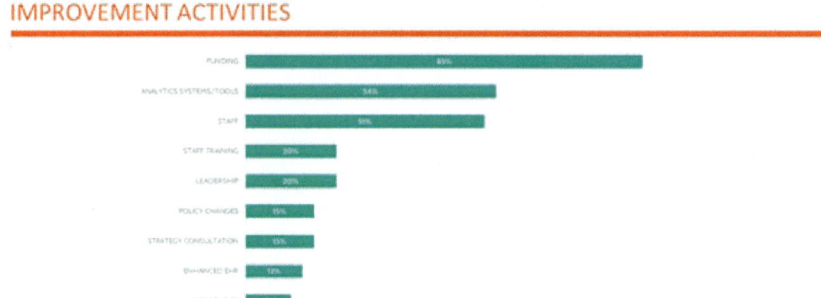

FIGURE 3-4 Additional resources needed for population health improvement activities.
NOTE: EHR = electronic health record.
SOURCES: Ramiah presentation, March 22, 2019; AEH, 2016; preliminary results as of July 5, 2016.

many of their peers did not know much about the work, and these executives did not have much internal credibility. Ramiah explained that the project team also learned that many of the population health executives had formerly been hospital chief operations officers or chief executive officers (CEOs) and were not trained in population health.

The project team's research led to some key findings about the role of a population health executive at essential hospitals. Internal and external core functions included leadership management, communication, collaboration, and measurement. With respect to the operating environment, there was variation among hospitals, with some being part of an accountable care organization risk-based model. Internal structure (where the population health activities were based and how they were dispersed) also varied among hospitals.

Ramiah noted that as a result of the survey findings, AEH recently released a Toolkit for Hiring and Evaluating Population Health Executives,[7] which describes who population health executives are, outlines what skill

---

[7] For more information about the Toolkit for Hiring and Evaluating Population Health Executives, see the webinar hosted by the Collaborative on Bridging Public Health, Health Care & Community at http://nationalacademies.org/hmd/Activities/PublicHealth/PopulationHealthImprovementRT/Action-Collaborative-Public-Health-Health-Care-Community (accessed May 10, 2021).

sets are needed, and provides a job description template for hospitals to use. The organization was also working with the directors of graduate medical education (GME) to incorporate population health activities into their training residency programs.

STATE OF PUBLIC HEALTH EDUCATION[8]

Laura Rasar King from CEPH spoke about the state of public health education in her remarks as a discussant. She began by providing background on CEPH, explaining that it is "the accrediting body for schools and programs in public health, established about 45 years ago as an independent accrediting body, recognized by the Department of Education. [The organization] accredits public health training programs from [the] baccalaureate level to the doctoral level."[9]

Public health education has grown significantly in the past several decades. As King noted, when the organization was established in 1974, it accredited 10 schools of public health, and as of the date of the workshop, there were 66 accredited schools of public health, 121 accredited public health programs, and 13 accredited baccalaureate programs not affiliated with a graduate public health program.

King described a couple of the transformations in public health education and training over the past decade. First, her organization identified core components of a bachelor's degree in public health, and students' interest in these programs is growing. She noted that the focus on baccalaureate public health programs was in response to concerns that some entities—particularly local public health departments in underserved areas—were unable to recruit enough master's-trained individuals. As of the date of the workshop, there were 79 accredited undergraduate programs in public health, and King noted that this number continues to grow. The required curriculum for a baccalaureate public health program incorporates concepts of population health as one of nine domains. Population health training includes basic processes, approaches, and interventions that identify and address major health needs and concerns, data collection and analysis, planning and assessment, and evaluation.

The second transformation is related to the Master of Public Health (M.P.H.) degree. As King explained, the M.P.H. degree changed very little in the first century since the Welch-Rose Report described it in 1915. However, CEPH reviewed the pertinent literature along with the PH

---

[8] This section summarizes information presented by Laura Rasar King from CEPH. The statements made are not endorsed or verified by the National Academies of Sciences, Engineering, and Medicine.

[9] More information about CEPH is available at https://ceph.org (accessed May 10, 2021).

WINS, the Council on Linkages competencies, and the National Board of Public Health Examiners Job Task Analysis. In 2016, the council issued revised criteria that "completely transformed what was expected in terms of public health education at the master's level." As King explained, the M.P.H. degree previously had five core courses: epidemiology, biostatistics, health services administration, environmental health, and social and behavioral sciences. Current M.P.H. programs are founded on 22 competencies and 8 domains, which are infused with population health, social determinants of health, and cultural competency. The eight domains are (1) evidence-based approaches, including data collection, analysis, and interpretation; (2) public health and health care systems; (3) planning and management, including budgeting and finance; (4) policy; (5) leadership, including visioning, strategic planning, negotiation, and mediation; (6) communication, both oral and written; (7) interprofessional practice; and (8) systems thinking. The council collected early data, which show that 84 percent of public health schools and programs have changed their core curricula, including the classes and class structure, to match these domains. The remaining 16 percent have kept the previous five core courses but changed the content within them.

LOCAL PUBLIC HEALTH WORKFORCE CONSIDERATIONS[10]

Kaye Bender from PHAB served as the second discussant and provided remarks regarding local public health workforce considerations. PHAB accredits governmental public health departments across the country. The 11-year-old organization recently launched an additional program for Army preventive medicine public health units and statewide vital records health statistics accreditation.[11]

Public health department accreditation standards are based on the framework of the 10 essential services of public health, which was selected, as Bender noted, because it was familiar to most public health departments. There are 12 domains, 10 of which are related directly to the 10 essential public health services, with 1 for management and 1 for governance.

Bender focused the remainder of her remarks on her organization's work related to workforce development and lessons learned. Bender noted that her organization began work with the following assumptions: (1) less

---

[10] This section summarizes information presented by Kaye Bender from PHAB. The statements made are not endorsed or verified by the National Academies of Sciences, Engineering, and Medicine.

[11] More information about PHAB is available at https://www.phaboard.org (accessed May 10, 2021).

than 10 percent of M.P.H. program graduates went into governmental public health; (2) as a result, most of the governmental public health workforce was not formally educated in public health; (3) government merit systems were an obstacle to workforce innovation and change; and (4) there was no standardized nationwide needs assessment approach, although this final point is no longer true with the development of the PH WINS.

There are two overarching standards in the domain related to workforce, the first from the recognition that less than 10 percent of M.P.H. program graduates went into governmental public health. To address this, health departments have been asked to partner with academic institutions to give students access to public health experiences to promote the development of future public health workers. Bender noted that most health departments do this, as long as there are schools or programs that teach public health content in their immediate geographic area.

The second standard is ensuring a competent workforce through assessing staff competencies, providing individual training and professional development, and creating a supportive work environment, which includes producing a workforce development plan. In the past, partners at the Association of State and Territorial Health Officials (ASTHO), the National Association of County and City Health Officials (NACCHO), the Public Health Foundation, and others have assisted health departments in assessing the needs of the workforce and developing a plan to address them. However, Bender noted that she agrees with Castrucci that the PH WINS eliminates the need for continued assessments, and the focus should be on plan development and implementation.

Bender closed her remarks by stating that health departments have made significant progress in addressing workforce issues, but she agrees with past speakers that there is much more work to be done. She noted that PHAB is in the process of refreshing its standards and measures in the area of workforce development.

PHYSICIAN EDUCATION AND HEALTH EQUITY[12]

The final discussant of the session was Lisa Howley from AAMC. She remarked on physician education and health equity. Howley began her comments by providing brief background on AAMC and its work related to the population health workforce.[13] It was founded in 1876

---

[12] This section summarizes information presented by Lisa Howley from AAMC. The statements made are not endorsed or verified by the National Academies of Sciences, Engineering, and Medicine.

[13] More information about AAMC and its programs is available at https://www.aamc.org (accessed May 10, 2021).

and is a nonprofit association "dedicated to transforming health care through medical education, research, and patient care."[14] Its mission is to serve and lead the academic medicine community for the health of all. Members include 154 U.S. medical schools, 17 Canadian medical schools, nearly 400 major teaching hospitals and health systems, including 51 Department of Veterans Affairs (VA) medical centers, and 80 academic societies. Through these institutions, AAMC serves more than 170,000 full-time faculty members, 90,000 medical students, 130,000 resident physicians, and 60,000 graduate students and postdoctoral researchers in biomedical sciences. Howley explained that as a member service organization, AAMC does not regulate practices, set standards, or conduct accreditations; it has a "supportive, informative, and developmental" relationship with its members.

Howley mentioned that AAMC is particularly dedicated to the issues of health equity, community, and population health. As an example, its most recent annual leadership forum was focused on community engagement to address health disparities. Howley acknowledged that reducing health disparities requires that medical schools and teaching hospitals "invest in building bidirectional trust, developing meaningful relationships, and understanding the historical perspectives of the community members that they serve." AAMC is actively engaged in population and public health research, clinical practice, and innovations. However, Howley's focus is medical education, so she provided additional examples within that area.

Howley noted that over the past few decades, higher education, including medicine, has shifted to a competency-based model. AAMC recently released new competencies, and quality improvement in patient safety and health equity is one of those five domains. The competencies were developed over an 18-month period with broad stakeholder input and community collaboration and are intended to support curricular design and assessment across the continuum of medical education for medical students, residents, and practicing physicians.

AAMC also recently partnered with the Provider Training and Education Workgroup led by Don Bradley and Bill Dietz, an ad hoc activity of the National Academies' Roundtable on Obesity Solutions. As Howley explained, the workgroup developed core interprofessional competencies for obesity prevention and management and is working to extend improvements in nutrition and physical activity education to health profession schools beyond medicine.

In addition, for more than 20 years, AAMC has had an interprofessional cooperative agreement with CDC focused on enhancing population

---

[14] See https://www.aamc.org/who-we-are (accessed May 10, 2021).

health education and providing experiential opportunities for medical, nursing, and public health students. A number of projects are being conducted under this cooperative agreement. One example is a free Web-based directory known as Public Health Pathways, which includes more than 200 domestic and international public health training opportunities across the education continuum and across professions. As another example, in 2019, AAMC published a monograph featuring lessons learned and best practices within GME residency programs for effectively teaching and modeling population health management in a primary care setting.

Additionally, AAMC hosted a national workshop in May 2019 for educational leaders from U.S. medical schools to advance medical education to combat opioid misuse. An additional initiative is the MedEdPORTAL, an open-access, peer-reviewed publication that promotes educational scholarship and the dissemination of teaching and educational resource materials, which AAMC co-sponsors with the American Dental Education Association. There is a collection focused on diversity, inclusion, and health equity that includes publications addressing topics such as food insecurity, community and home violence, cultural humility, obesity care, homelessness, and school health.

Within its Scientific Affairs Division, AAMC has an initiative titled Accelerating Health Equity: Advancing Through Discovery, the mission of which is to identify, evaluate, and disseminate effective and replicable AAMC member institution practices that are improving community health and reducing health inequities.[15]

In closing, Howley emphasized that she believes that improving population health is an important part of a physician's responsibilities and "requires an educational program that is competency based and designed to mutually benefit the local needs of the academic health system and the communities within which they serve."

DISCUSSION

As session moderator, Meadows opened the audience discussion by highlighting some key takeaways and asking the speakers two questions: whether the right people are being targeted for additional training in public health and what is being done to create a supportive work environment in local government that embraces population health and health equity.

Bender responded by providing anecdotes from her 40 years of experience in public health. Bender mentioned she is aware of many courses

---

[15] See https://www.aamc.org/what-we-do/mission-areas/medical-research/rocc/sponsored-award-programs/donaghue-grants (accessed May 10, 2021).

targeting public health leaders and is unsure whether this training is directed at the appropriate level. Bender noted that having well-trained leaders is important but that these leaders often do not stay in their positions very long, particularly at the state level.

In response to Meadows's second question, Bender answered that she believes leadership's actions matter. She noted that she is referring to leadership as more than a single health department leader. As she explained, "You get a progressive, well educated in the whole arena of managing the public health department leader, who surrounds him- or herself with other leaders who are interested in quality improvement, interested in health equity, interested in being innovative, then you see that health department make an almost dramatic shift." Bender added that the importance of leadership is particularly evident after a dynamic leader leaves and there is a loss of that type of leadership.

Ramiah added that she agrees regarding the importance of leadership for population health. She noted that most of the success stories with essential hospitals come from places where the CEO and population health executive are coordinated and aware of each other's priorities. Ramiah spoke of the importance of this "dual leadership," which comes from "peer pressure, ... environmental changes, and ... motivation that needs to get to the board and the CEO," rather than skills or training.

In response to the question as to whether training is happening at the right level, Castrucci answered based on his experience in government public health, pointing out that training is often only offered to people with certain titles or at a certain level. He noted that state public health commissioners may not have prior experience within government or public health and questioned how this may impact the governmental public health workforce they are tasked with leading.

Sagar Shah from the American Planning Association asked Castrucci whether his organization had assessed any geographic patterns in the public health workers who intend to leave their organization and whether any particular areas of the country are in crisis. Castrucci responded by stating that the PH WINS needs to improve the question on where potentially departing workers intend to go. He explained that there are geographical differences; however, because the PH WINS is conducted in partnership with ASTHO, NACCHO, and the Big Cities Health Coalition, regional and state data are available, but there is an agreement not to release individual state-level data without the permission of the state health official.

Anna Ricklin from the Fairfax County Health Department in Virginia asked panelists to comment on the data point Castrucci presented that most local public health workers support health equity but are not familiar with or supportive of the concept of health in all policies. She asked panelists for their thoughts on what can be done to shift the culture. Castrucci responded that he was not surprised that local public health departments are not engaged in health in all policies because they are not funded to do so. He suggested that national government public health agencies, such as CDC, and national organizations, such as ASTHO, NACCHO, and the American Public Health Association, determine that health in all policies is important and provide training on how state and local public health agencies can implement them. Bender agreed, emphasizing the importance of removing silos in categorical program funding and noting that with funding cuts, health department staff often work to protect the funds for their program.

Ron Bialek from the Public Health Foundation asked whether there are further plans to support public health departments in addressing needs and gaps, based on factors such as current workforce composition and organizational priorities. Meadows clarified that given the topic of the workshop, the focus should be on addressing needs and gaps specifically to support population health. Bender responded by explaining that PHAB asks health departments to consider how to align their workforce development plan and implementation with their overall strategic plan, which they have been asked to align with their community health improvement plan.

Maryjoan Ladden from the Robert Wood Johnson Foundation explained that the foundation has been working on population health preparation in nursing and is moving toward expanding it to all health professionals. She asked the panel "how well they think population health competencies and capabilities are integrated into accreditation standards and curricula across medicine, nursing, social work, and other health professions." King responded that with respect to training in public health, there was a report by the Association of Schools & Programs of Public Health called *Population Health Across All Professions* (ASPPH, 2015). As another example, King explained that the Association of Specialized and Professional Accreditors—the membership association for accrediting bodies in all professions, including the health professions—worked on a task force a few years ago on a professional doctorate among all the health professions. She noted that population health was one of the areas that was common in the professional doctorate. Points made by the speakers in this section are highlighted below (see Box 3-1).

BOX 3-1
Points Made by Individual Speakers and Participants

- While there is a high level of job satisfaction in the governmental public health workforce, many workers plan to leave their jobs in the near future. Other than retirement, top reasons for departure include inadequate pay, lack of advancement, workplace environment, low job satisfaction, and lack of support. (Castrucci)
- Essential hospitals are addressing social determinants of health both inside their own walls and in their communities. (Ramiah)
- Two major changes in public health education and training over the past decade are an expansion in the number of baccalaureate public health programs and a transformation of the M.P.H. degree to increase focus on population health, social determinants of health, and cultural competency. (King)
- Less than 10 percent of M.P.H. program graduates go into governmental public health. Therefore, most of the governmental public health workforce is not formally trained in public health. (Bender)
- Actions by leadership are particularly important in creating an environment that supports population health and health equity. (Bender, Ramiah)
- Success stories within hospitals often occur when the views of the population health executive and chief executive officer are in sync. (Ramiah)
- Training in public health is often directed toward individuals in leadership positions. (Castrucci) There are mixed views regarding whether this is the most appropriate audience. (Bender, Castrucci)

NOTE: This list is the rapporteurs' summary of the main points made by individual speakers and participants (noted in parentheses) and does not reflect any consensus among workshop participants or endorsement by the National Academies of Sciences, Engineering, and Medicine participants, or endorsement by the National Academies.

4

The Community Health Workforce

COMMUNITY HEALTH WORKER PANEL[1]

The session moderator, Karen Murphy from Geisinger, opened the session by explaining that it would have three components. The first portion would be a panel of community health workers (CHWs), who are "on the ground" directly touching people's lives. The second portion would be four presentations related to CHW workforce issues, and the third portion would be a discussion with workshop participants. The CHW panel included the following individuals:

- Shanteny Jackson, Richmond City Health District and Virginia Community Health Worker Association (VACHWA)
- Kevin Jordan, Damien Ministries and Maryland Community Health Worker Advisory Committee
- Orson Brown, Penn Center for Community Health Workers
- Adriana Rodriguez Palacios, Oregon Community Health Worker Association (ORCHWA)

---

[1] This section summarizes information presented by the following CHWs on the CHW panel: Shanteny Jackson, Richmond City Health District and VACHWA; Kevin Jordan, Damien Ministries and Maryland Community Health Worker Advisory Committee; Orson Brown, Penn Center for Community Health Workers; and Adriana Rodriguez Palacios, ORCHWA. The statements made are not endorsed or verified by the National Academies of Sciences, Engineering, and Medicine.

Karen Murphy opened by asking the panel members what they see as the role of a CHW and how it intersects with the health care delivery system.

Shanteny Jackson explained that while the specific role varies by community, standard activities include navigation, outreach, advocacy, and education. She clarified that "navigation" refers to navigation within the health care system. "Outreach" means connecting to the services available in the community. "Advocacy" involves empowering clients to be self-sufficient and address barriers. "Education" refers to strategies that transform barriers into advantages and allow progress toward achieving the goals of thriving individuals and thriving communities.

Kevin Jordan answered by stating that he sees CHWs as the liaison between the community and the clinical or health care setting. CHWs are members of the community they are trying to reach. Their goals are to engage other community members, bring them into a clinical setting, and link them to health services. Jordan noted that CHWs address a continuum of care and provided an example based on his experience addressing HIV/AIDS. First, CHWs conduct outreach and education regarding HIV and sexually transmitted infections (STIs). Next, they work to bring people in for an initial walk-in screening using rapid HIV testing. Depending on that test result, CHWs try to link the person to a clinical setting that offers a "gold standard" HIV test. CHWs support members of the community, communicate with both medical and nonmedical case managers, and help to ensure that people show up to appointments. Jordan explained that medical and nonmedical case managers at the entity where he works have said that CHWs are helpful in providing support, increasing retention, and improving medication adherence.

Orson Brown added that an important role of CHWs is to bridge gaps in the health sector. He noted that many patients in the communities they serve may mistrust or misunderstand medical professionals or feel that they are not being heard. The role of the CHW is to get to know patients and partner with them to develop an achievable plan for meeting health goals. Brown noted that his organization, the Penn Center for Community Health Workers, has seen success from CHWs helping people first to understand the barriers preventing them from attending doctors' appointments, and then to develop a plan for addressing them.

Murphy next asked the panelists what they see as key elements of success for a CHW. Adriana Rodriguez Palacios responded by stating that, most importantly, a CHW has to be a trusted member of the community who can identify the real needs of that community. Brown agreed with Palacios and added that appropriate training and oversight are also important for CHWs' success. He pointed out that CHWs can easily get overwhelmed or burned out by the work, and support from management is important in overcoming this.

Jackson also added that it is important for CHWs to be part of a multidisciplinary team that includes clinical staff. Each team member has a unique role, and the team-based approach facilitates addressing multiple challenges that a person may have. For example, at the Richmond City Health District where Jackson works, team members include a resource center specialist, CHW, nurse practitioner, and public health nurse. The resource center specialist welcomes and registers the clients and refers them to the CHW if any issues cannot be addressed initially. The CHW connects with the clients before they see a health care provider to address any initial questions, which allows the health care provider to focus on their medical needs. Next, a client may reconnect with the CHW for help with navigating to a particular service or addressing other social needs.

Murphy next asked how the CHW profession is growing or changing over time. Jordan responded that he has been a CHW for 5 years, and in that time, he has noticed researchers and public health officials dedicating more attention to CHWs and their role. For example, in Prince George's County, Maryland, where he lives, a workgroup was established in 2014 to advise on the types of training and workforce development that CHWs need. In 2018, Maryland passed a bill to create a CHW advisory committee on trainings and certifications. As another example, in the District of Columbia the Department of Health recently began considering what a CHW structure might look like and invited community members and other stakeholders to participate in discussions. Jordan added that there is a trend toward developing a certification for CHWs because other health professions, such as nursing and social work, require certifications, which provide increased recognition and credibility. Some states, such as Virginia, have made progress toward requiring certifications for CHWs. Jordan noted that Maryland and the District of Columbia are also moving in that direction, but there are no requirements yet.

STANDARDIZED, SCALABLE, AND EFFECTIVE COMMUNITY HEALTH WORKER PROGRAMS TO IMPROVE POPULATION HEALTH

Shreya Kangovi from the Division of General Internal Medicine, the Perelman School of Medicine, and the Penn Center for Community Health Workers at the University of Pennsylvania began her presentation by sharing a story of a patient[2] who had suffered childhood trauma and spent time incarcerated as an adult. When he was released, he struggled with estrangement from his family and difficulty finding housing. He lived in an aban-

---

[2] This section summarizes information presented by Shreya Kangovi from the Penn Center for Community Health Workers. The statements made are not endorsed or verified by the National Academies of Sciences, Engineering, and Medicine.

doned store without heat and tried to take his life nine times in a 6-month period. He was hospitalized each time and met with a psychiatrist and social worker but ended up in the same situation. During the final hospitalization, this patient met a CHW named Cheryl, who took the time to get to know him as a person. She asked him when he had last laughed. He responded that he had not wholeheartedly laughed in 27 years, and the last time was when he was out bowling. When he was discharged from the hospital, Cheryl and another CHW took him bowling, which reminded him that there could be joy in life. After that outing, CHWs worked to get him the behavioral health, primary care, and housing support he needed. However, it was their creative and "outside-the-box" thinking that was successful in getting him the help he needed. Kangovi explained that CHWs live the "health for all" motto, which often involves more than just the health care system.

Kangovi defined CHWs as individuals who come from within and are demographic mirrors of the communities they serve. They are uniquely altruistic, or "natural helpers." CHWs differ from navigators, health coaches, and care coordinators, although they perform all of these roles at times. The concept of a CHW has existed for at least two centuries, gaining and losing prominence over time. Kangovi pointed out that, historically, CHW programs have failed more than they have succeeded. She noted five reasons, according to a global review of the implementation science literature. The first reason is that often the wrong people are hired for the job, leading to turnover rates of 50–77 percent cited in the published literature (Nkonki et al., 2011). Improved recruitment strategies, behavioral screening, and case-based interviews could help address this issue. The second reason is lack of standardized infrastructure, such as supervision, management of caseload, and processes to ensure safety of CHWs in the field. Kangovi noted that there is often no intervention model for CHWs to follow. She suggested that manuals for CHWs, managers, and program directors could help to address this issue. The third and fourth reasons relate to lack of balance between clinical integration and retaining grassroots identity. The final reason is the lack of scientific evidence regarding the field of social determinants broadly and CHW programs specifically. Kangovi noted that most studies on the impact of CHWs have been pre–post studies with limitations that overestimate the effect of CHW programs and create a hype that she sees as damaging in the long term.

Kangovi provided suggestions for elevating the CHW role by systematically addressing historical limitations. To improve hiring, organizational and psychological principles have been used to develop hiring algorithms unique to the CHW workforce, which has reduced turnover. To create standardized work practices, easy-to-read manuals have been written and refined with input from CHWs. Manuals have been developed for CHWs, supervisors, and program directors. Trainings and certifications have also been produced for all levels, including CHWs, supervisors, and program directors. Kangovi developed a software application for CHW workflow, documentation, and reporting, noting that CHWs often document their engagement in a patient's electronic medical record, pulling them further into the medical model. She added that the software was designed because there is a need for technology to support a CHW workflow that goes beyond screening and referral.

Kangovi further emphasized the need for more research on whether the CHW model is working and how it can best operate with the goal of improving population health. She mentioned that there have been three randomized controlled trials (RCTs) assessing the effectiveness of the Individualized Management for Patient-Centered Targets (IMPaCT) worker model. Kangovi's presentation highlighted that these studies, published in the *American Journal of Public Health* (Kangovi et al., 2017) and the *Journal of the American Medical Association* (Kangovi et al., 2014), have shown consistent improvements in outcomes in some areas, including a 65 percent decrease in cost and 12 and 16 percent increases in access and quality, respectively.

Kangovi stated that programs often overestimate return on investment (ROI) because these estimates come from pre–post studies that are often limited by regression to the mean. Based on the three RCTs, Kangovi's team has estimated the ROI for the IMPaCT model to be $2:1. This validated and favorable ROI has fueled rapid expansion of the program within Philadelphia and across the country. The Penn Center has served 10,000 patients in the Philadelphia region and disseminated tools, training, and technical assistance to 1,000 organizations nationwide.

Kangovi explained that the Penn Center is also working with accreditation bodies, such as the National Committee for Quality Assurance, to consider CHW program-level accreditation, which shifts the burden of accreditation and training from the individual CHW to the program employing the CHWs. Kangovi closed her presentation by highlighting important issues to consider, including the tension between individual versus program accreditation, the role of science in evaluation of CHW programs, and a career ladder for the CHW workforce.

COMMUNITY HEALTH WORKER WORKFORCE DEVELOPMENT AND THE OREGON COMMUNITY HEALTH WORKERS ASSOCIATION

The next presentation by Noelle Wiggins from ORCHWA provided participants with background on the association and how it operates.[3,4]

---

[3] This section summarizes information presented by Noelle Wiggins from ORCHWA. The statements made are not endorsed or verified by the National Academies of Sciences, Engineering, and Medicine.

[4] More information about ORCHWA and its initiatives is available at http://www.orchwa.org (accessed May 10, 2021).

This included an overview of its origins, its funding, how it interacts with Oregon's coordinated care organizations (CCOs), and its work in evaluation and research with and about CHWs and in CHW training and workforce development.

Wiggins began by sharing ORCHWA's definition of CHWs: "trusted community members who participate in capacitation, or empowering training, so that they can promote health in their own communities…. Communities can be defined by race/ethnicity, geography, age, sexual orientation, disability status, other factors, or a combination of factors." ORCHWA also supports a longer definition[5] of a CHW developed by the American Public Health Association, with which they have been involved since the 1990s. ORCHWA's CHW definition is complemented by its understanding of CHW and *promotor/promotora* history. She noted that this model grew out of natural helping and healing mechanisms that have existed in all communities since the beginning of human history. CHW models became formalized in areas where people were systematically denied health care and the conditions necessary for good health. Therefore, the CHW model is dedicated to increasing health equity.

As background on ORCHWA's history, Wiggins explained that Oregon has had a history of successful CHW and *promotor/promotora* programs since the 1960s. Foundational CHW programs in the state have included the community health representative program founded at the Confederated Tribes of the Umatilla Indian Reservation in 1967, outreach worker programs that began in county health departments during the HIV/AIDS crisis in the 1980s, and the El Niño Sano ("The Healthy Child") program that was started in 1988 at La Clinica del Cariño in Hood River, Oregon. Wiggins's first job with CHWs in the United States was as the program director at El Niño Sano.

In 1994, *promotores* from El Niño Sano, which functioned for 10 years, helped organize the first statewide CHW, *promotor*, and *promotora* organization under the auspices of the Oregon Public Health Association. In 2011, CHWs and allies in the state of Oregon became aware that policy was being created about them as part of health care reform, and while individual CHWs were involved, the profession did not have a unified

---

[5] A CHW is a frontline public health worker who is a trusted member of and/or has an unusually close understanding of the community served. This trusting relationship enables the worker to serve as a liaison, link, or intermediary between health and social services and the community to facilitate access to services and improve the quality and cultural competence of service delivery. A CHW also builds individual and community capacity by increasing health knowledge and self-sufficiency through a range of activities such as outreach, community education, informal counseling, social support, and advocacy. See https://www.apha.org/apha-communities/member-sections/community-health-workers (accessed May 10, 2021).

and organized voice. With funding from the Northwest Regional Primary Care Association, two leadership development workshops were organized in two regions of Oregon. These served as the jumping off point for ORCHWA, with the mission to "serve as a unified voice to empower and advocate for CHWs and our communities."[6] ORCHWA held its first meeting in November 2011.

Initially, ORCHWA did not have any funding and was supported by in-kind donations from the Oregon Latino Health Coalition and Community Capacitation Center at the Multnomah County health department. After a few small to moderate grants, in 2017, ORCHWA received a 2-year, $3 million investment from Health Share of Oregon, the state's largest CCO. As Wiggins explained, in Oregon, a CCO is a group of health systems and provider groups that apply to the state to be funded to serve Medicaid beneficiaries in a given region. As of the date of the workshop, ORCHWA had more than 13 funding sources, including grants, contracts, and fee-for-service arrangements, providing an annual budget of more than $3 million, which Wiggins noted is a large budget for a CHW association.

Wiggins highlighted the importance of Health Share's investment, the purpose of which was to support ORCHWA in building infrastructure that would allow it to serve as a broker between health systems that want to access the services of CHWs and *promotores* and community-based organizations that employ these individuals. Wiggins sees several benefits to this arrangement. First, she believes that CHW programs need to be supported by health care reform and the funding that comes with it. Second, CHWs in culturally specific organizations are often supported to maintain cultural world views and cultural approaches to health. Third, CHWs in community-based organizations may be better able to play a full range of roles, including organizer and advocate. Wiggins also hopes that this arrangement will increase salaries for CHWs in community-based organizations.

When the infrastructure is fully developed, ORCHWA will offer certification training for CHWs and their supervisors, have an online case management platform, and provide research and evaluation services. Wiggins explained that ORCHWA was also developing a contract with Kaiser Permanente and pursuing contracts with other health systems.

Wiggins next described ORCHWA's training and workforce development programs. Assessment of training needs happens both formally and informally. A regional and statewide assessment serves as the formal mechanism. ORCHWA employs CHWs and convenes three collaboratives, including CHWs, their supervisors, and funders, which also allows it to receive

---

[6] See https://www.orchwa.org/about-us/mission-statement (accessed May 10, 2021).

regular feedback informally. The methodology and philosophy ORCHWA uses for CHW training is Popular/People's Education, which is associated with Brazilian educator and political theorist Paolo Freire and based on the idea that the people most affected by inequities are the experts about their own experience. ORCHWA and its community-based organization partners also provide cross-cultural, culturally specific initial and ongoing training.

Wiggins concluded by explaining that ORCHWA is committed to conducting research and evaluation with and about CHWs to contribute to the body of credible evidence in partnership with CHWs using a community-based participatory research and evaluation framework. ORCHWA is also committed to building the skills of CHWs as researchers, including supporting them to obtain more formal education when they so desire.

COMMUNITY HEALTH WORKER TRAINING AND THE FUTURE OF THE PROFESSION[7]

Michael Rhein and Dwyan Monroe from the Institute for Public Health Innovation (IPHI) spoke about where and how CHWs fit into the health sector, CHW training needs, the ROI of employing CHWs, the state of CHWs and CHW associations, and changes to the role with changes in the health care system and an increased focus on population health.

Rhein explained that as the public health institute serving the District of Columbia, Maryland, and Virginia for the past decade, IPHI has the mission of leading innovative solutions to public health issues in the region and working at a systems level to address workforce development, advocacy, capacity building, convening, and leading the development of effective interventions.[8] As Rhein described, the community health workforce is not a panacea, but it is an integral component of a strategy to address health equity. IPHI has trained more than 600 CHWs in its region in the past 10 years and is leading conversations around scope of practice and certification, providing resources for demonstration projects and pilots, and conducting evaluations. The organization is also working to advocate for the CHW profession and ensure that CHWs and their partners have a "seat at the table" where decisions about them are being made.

Rhein highlighted that as a result of work by IPHI and partners, the District of Columbia, Maryland, and Virginia have all worked collaboratively with CHWs to define scope of practice, core competencies,

---

[7] This section summarizes information presented by Michael Rhein and Dwyan Monroe from IPHI. The statements made are not endorsed or verified by the National Academies of Sciences, Engineering, and Medicine.

[8] More information about IPHI and its initiatives is available at https://www.institutephi.org (accessed May 10, 2021).

and training requirements, and progress has been made toward CHW certification. In addition, employment opportunities for CHWs have been created and integrated into the business models for hospitals, Medicaid-managed care organizations, and health departments. CHWs have been involved as leaders and advocates in this work.

Despite significant progress, Rhein noted several areas where there is still work to be done. First, he sees a need to address the lack of awareness, understanding, and appreciation of the CHW role and more fully integrate them into multi-disciplinary teams. Second, he highlighted an ongoing tension between CHWs' community roots and the move toward increased professionalism and certification (and the health system's call for this). To manage this, IPHI advocates for voluntary certification, and Rhein noted that certification and training needs may vary depending on the community and the CHW's scope of work. He believes it is important for the CHW role to be owned by the community and for there to be respect for its "lay" history. Rhein also sees the need for more sustainable financing mechanisms, such as including CHWs in value-based contracts and Medicaid managed care approaches. Rhein also suggested that health care providers, health departments, and other entities that employ CHWs see them as part of their business model, including the ROI, rather than simply funding them through grants.

Monroe began by explaining that she is a former CHW with 25 years of experience. Monroe noted the importance of understanding that lived experience is half the experience that CHWs bring, and the training that is provided is intended to address particular diseases and issues and give CHWs an opportunity to become part of the health professional workforce. The training also provides access to employer-financed education for people who might not otherwise have that opportunity, through mechanisms such as apprenticeships. This removes an educational barrier to recruiting the right people for the CHW role. Monroe explained that IPHI, for example, offers a $100 course that addresses CHW core skills and competencies and provides basic health information, including an overview of all major chronic diseases, mental health issues, and trauma-informed care. IPHI also promotes health equity through a 2-day perspective transformation training for CHWs that addresses prejudice, race, and the CHW role.

Monroe noted that IPHI also supports team integration, and she added that there is interest among organizations employing CHWs in providing initial training for CHWs but less interest in team-based trainings that include the CHW, supervisor, and other team members and provide an opportunity to discuss issues related to triage and workflow. She suggested that when problems are reported with a CHW, they may stem from team-based issues.

Related to CHW advocacy, Monroe explained that there are about 45 CHW associations or networks and an entity called Unity that hosts a national CHW conference. These organizations unite CHWs and give them a "voice." She suggested that, as with nurses and other health professionals who may seek ongoing professional development to meet accreditation requirements, CHWs would benefit from outside workshops, trainings, and conferences that address and support their critical role.

POPULATION HEALTH WORKFORCE SUPPORT FOR DISADVANTAGED AREAS PROGRAM[9]

Katie Wunderlich from the Maryland Health Services Cost Review Commission presented on the challenges of integrating payment for CHWs into the business model of delivering health care across the care spectrum. She also described how Maryland has promoted the use of CHWs through regulatory processes and health care system initiatives, including financing mechanisms for hospitals and other community-based organizations. Although CHW services are often not reimbursed in a fee-for-service payment model, Maryland has a unique value-based approach that allows hospitals to use revenue to pay for CHWs' services and other services that promote community and population health.

As background, the Maryland Health Services Cost Review Commission is a state agency responsible for setting hospital rates throughout the state. The agency also leads a statewide health care delivery transformation focused on breaking down siloed sites of care and coordinating care across the health care setting. As Wunderlich explained, the state's "total cost of care model" that has resulted from this is intended to coordinate patient care across both hospital and nonhospital settings, improve health outcomes, and constrain cost growth. Hospitals are compensated using a value-based payment system, which allows for health and social services that promote population health to be incorporated into and paid for by the hospital system. The model is provider led and focused on sustaining rural hospitals. There has also been a focus on population health improvement, using incentives to address the health of the population the hospital serves, break down silos, and coordinate care across the spectrum. To that end, one specific goal is incorporating CHWs into the health care delivery system.

In 2015, the Maryland Health Services Cost Review Commission approved a 3-year, $10 million initiative for hospitals to hire and train

---

[9] This section summarizes information presented by Katie Wunderlich from the Maryland Health Services Cost Review Commission. The statements made are not endorsed or verified by the National Academies of Sciences, Engineering, and Medicine.

workers from areas of high economic disparities and unemployment. Participating hospitals had to match half the funds and hire, train, and support workers to fill new positions focused on improving population health and meeting other goals identified in the total cost of care model. As Wunderlich described, there were two main goals of the program. The first was to provide employment opportunities in disadvantaged communities, as stable employment is an important social determinant of health. The second was to improve population health in Maryland through workforce investments.

Funding was provided through this initiative for Garrett County and for the Baltimore Population Health Workforce Collaborative. The Baltimore Collaborative was the larger of the two and involved 9 hospitals with a goal of hiring 208 total CHWs, peer recovery specialists, certified nursing assistants, and geriatric nursing assistants by fiscal year (FY) 2019. The program was renewed, and funding will continue to support training and hiring through June 2022. Other key program partners included the Baltimore Alliance for Careers in Healthcare, which served as a training coordinator and intermediary with the hospital systems; Turnaround Tuesday, which provided support with recruiting, essential skills training, and wraparound services for workers; and CHW, nursing assistant, and peer recovery specialist organizations, which provided technical training for workers in these professions.

Wunderlich presented data on program outcomes. As of June 2018, 114 workers were trained and hired, including 73 CHWs. The training and hiring will continue through FY 2022. Patient care activities that were possible as a result included care coordination, health education and health system navigation, companion care and patient escort, transitional care, peer recovery, and linking to community services. Services were focused on a diverse patient population, concentrating on high-use and high-risk Medicare patients.

Wunderlich concluded by sharing some insights and lessons learned. First, there was a slow start, as it took time for hospitals to implement the idea of using their rate-setting system dollars for CHWs and for a collaborative to be established among Baltimore hospitals. There is still work to be done to reach the initial goal of training and hiring 208 workers. Second, community partnerships have been vital to recruiting, retaining, and providing wraparound services for workers to address retention. Another insight was the challenge in quantifying the impact or ROI of one CHW embedded in a hospital's larger population health initiatives. Anecdotal evidence provided support for renewing the program. Another goal for the program and similar ones is to provide upward mobility for workers in the hospital delivery system and larger health care system.

DISCUSSION

Following the presentations, there was an opportunity for members of the audience to ask questions of the CHW panelists and session presenters. Terry Allan from the Cuyahoga County Health Department in Greater Cleveland opened the session by asking the speakers what resources might be available for CHWs and nonprofit organizations that have relationships in the community and want to develop an agency to run their own business, as either a CHW or an organization employing CHWs, respectively. He noted that he has worked with CHWs and community-based organizations that could use support with business and back office operations.

Rhein responded that he sees a need for large institutions and government agencies to employ community members while also supporting smaller community-based organizations through authentic business partnerships. Large institutions provide an opportunity for CHWs to be members of integrated health care teams. CHWs in these positions can also help large organizations establish relationships with and reach deep into communities. Large institutions can also address economic opportunity as a determinant of health through CHW job creation and investment in communities. Rhein sees an indispensable role for grassroots community-based organizations that are themselves a way to reach into communities. He suggested that large institutions both hire community members as staff and form meaningful business relationships with community-based organizations that have traditionally had peers on their staff and have trust-based relationships with the community.

Wiggins added that ORCHWA contracted with CCOs so that individual community-based organizations would not have to do so. With this arrangement, ORCHWA is the broker between community-based organizations and the large health care institutions, providing the contracting capacity, relationships, training for CHWs and supervisors, support for creating job descriptions and recruitment, and evaluations of program impact.

Kangovi pointed out that there could be tension between the goals of workforce development and of improving population health. Using a firefighting analogy, she asked whether the goal is training firefighters or putting out fires. She suggested that the goal is putting out fires (i.e., improving population health), because if the goal is workforce development, the investment may or may not be effective in achieving the ultimate goal of improving population health. Kangovi also noted that partnerships with communities are often operationalized as partnerships with community-based organizations, the leadership of which may not represent those community members intended to benefit from the initiative.

Palacios also reiterated the importance of training for other team members who work with CHWs on how best to integrate CHWs into the workflow and the roles they can play outside the health care setting. She noted that one activity she did as a CHW was to collect signatures in support of sidewalks and lighting to improve the community's safety. She stated that while there may not be a billing code for this type of work in a health care setting, it is an important component of a CHW's job.

Kevin Barnett from the Public Health Institute and the California Health Workforce Alliance added three points for discussion. First, he suggested that CHW training programs be certified rather than CHWs themselves, explaining that many of the best CHWs with whom he has worked in California are undocumented and lack a high school diploma. Program certification allowed the medical community to be confident in the scope of the CHW training to supplement workers' lived experience and prepare them to work in health care teams. Second, Barnett pointed to the need to educate mainstream organizations regarding the benefits of hiring CHWs. Third, he highlighted the potential for the Pathways Community HUB Model of CHW engagement (PCHI, 2019), which is similar to ORCHWA's model of engaging CHWs through a nonprofit organization that partners with all of the payers and providers in an area. Barnett noted that this model allows CHWs to retain their agency and move beyond individual patient care management to broader population health improvement.

Wiggins responded to Barnett's third point about the Pathways model by suggesting that it be considered a method of evaluating the work rather than a payment model. Kangovi added that she supports Pathways as a way to bring health and social services organizations together, often using the same technology platform, to monitor the many health and social needs of a single individual. She noted that the CHW is the "human element" that can help the person address a spectrum of needs.

Kangovi also suggested that a successful CHW program involves both infrastructure and training. She recommended that a larger goal could be to develop a successful CHW program ecosystem that could be replicated and implemented anywhere in the United States. Wiggins phrased this as "spreading the CHW paradigm, which is community focused, [is] nonhierarchical, and values life experience, throughout the health system and dominant culture systems."

Sagar Shah from the American Planning Association asked how planners can help to train and support CHWs. Jackson responded that partners outside the health sector can support CHWs by establishing relationships and including CHWs' perspectives on committees and subcommittees where decisions are being made. Points made by the speakers in this section are highlighted below (see Box 4-1).

BOX 4-1
Points Made by Individual Speakers and Participants

- Community health worker (CHW) roles include community member education and empowerment, navigation within the health care system, and advocacy on behalf of the community's interests. (Brown, Jackson, Jordan)
- CHWs are to be trusted members of the communities they serve. (Brown, Kangovi, Monroe, Palacios)
- CHWs are most effective when part of a multi-disciplinary team that includes other health professionals. (Jackson, Monroe, Rhein)
- Training for CHWs could include training for their supervisors and other team members on how CHWs can best be employed within the team. (Monroe, Palacios)
- The limited number of randomized controlled trials on the impact of CHW programs shows mixed results. Potential reasons for lack of success include poor hiring practices, lack of standardized infrastructure, lack of balance between clinical integration and retaining grassroots identity, and lack of scientific evidence regarding the field of social determinants broadly and CHW programs specifically. (Kangovi)
- An ongoing tension exists between CHWs' community roots and the move toward increased professionalism and certification. (Barnett, Kangovi, Rhein)
- While workforce development and population health goals may seem aligned, there may be tension regarding which outcome is the ultimate goal. (Kangovi)
- Value-based payment systems for hospitals, such as Maryland's "total cost of care" model, allow health and social services that promote population health to be incorporated into and paid for by the hospital system. (Wunderlich)

NOTE: This list is the rapporteurs' summary of the main points made by individual speakers and participants (noted in parentheses) and does not reflect any consensus among workshop participants or endorsement by the National Academies of Sciences, Engineering, and Medicine.

5

Cross-Sector Workforce: National and Local Examples

Session moderator Gary Gunderson from the Wake Forest Baptist Medical Center, also representing Stakeholder Health, opened by providing a brief background on the session. It featured speakers from entities and organizations promoting population health by supporting other sectors in their efforts to incorporate a population health perspective into their missions, activities, and programs.

TRAIN LEARNING NETWORK AND COMPETENCIES FOR POPULATION HEALTH PROFESSIONALS[1]

Ron Bialek from the Public Health Foundation (PHF) outlined a two-part presentation. First, he gave an overview of the TrainingFinder Real-time Affiliate-Integrated Network (TRAIN) Learning Network, which has evolved from a narrow focus on governmental public health to one that is applicable to a broader range of health professionals, volunteers, and others.[2] Bialek then discussed the recently developed competencies for population health professionals.

Bialek explained that the mission of PHF is to improve public health and population health practice to support healthier communities.[3] He

---

[1] This section summarizes information presented by Ron Bialek from PHF. The statements made are not endorsed or verified by the National Academies of Sciences, Engineering, and Medicine.

[2] More information about the TRAIN Learning Network and its courses is available at https://www.train.org/main/welcome (accessed May 10, 2021).

[3] More information about PHF is available at http://www.phf.org/Pages/default.aspx (accessed May 10, 2021).

added that workforce development is key to that mission. He described that one of the organization's strategic goals was recently changed from "create opportunities for public health and health care alignment" to "create opportunities for cross-sector alignment," reflecting that addressing population health and community health involves more than the public health and health care sectors.

Fifteen years ago, Bialek added, PHF created the TRAIN Learning Network in response to a need from state and local public health departments to find, access, and track training opportunities. The network has grown to more than 1.8 million users with 10 million courses completed. The network offers 4,300 free courses delivered by more than 3,000 providers. Current users include about half of the governmental public workforce (263,250 people in public health agencies), about 600,000 people in health care, and about 450,000 people in private industry, nonprofit organizations, and other industries. There are also users in other government agencies, including transportation and behavioral health, and other sectors, including construction companies, places of worship, renewable energy companies, and brokerage firms.

The top jobs of TRAIN's users in public health and health care include nurses, emergency responders, public health and health care administrators, health officials, and frontline workers (see Figure 5-1).

Outside of public health and health care, the top TRAIN user roles are emergency responders, volunteers, management, and students. Students may receive non-degree-oriented training through the system that supplements their formal education (see Figure 5-2).

TRAIN addresses issues such as general public health, emergency preparedness, planning and policy, budgeting, and grants management. Bialek highlighted some examples of specific population health training topics, such as where to find and how to use data, healthy homes, food insecurity, principles of building construction, creating safe buildings, and

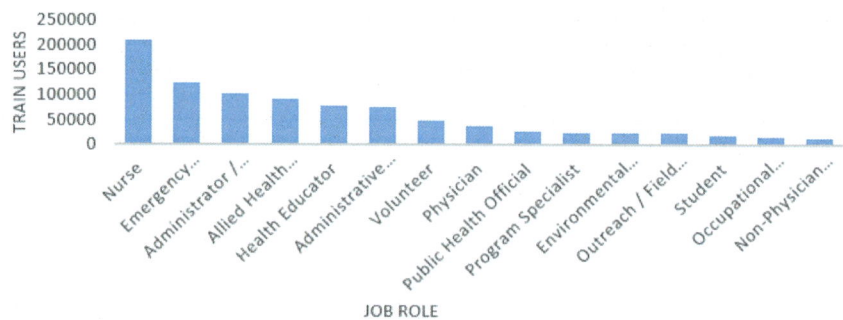

FIGURE 5-1 Top 15 job roles for TRAIN users in public health and health care.
SOURCE: Bialek presentation, March 22, 2019.

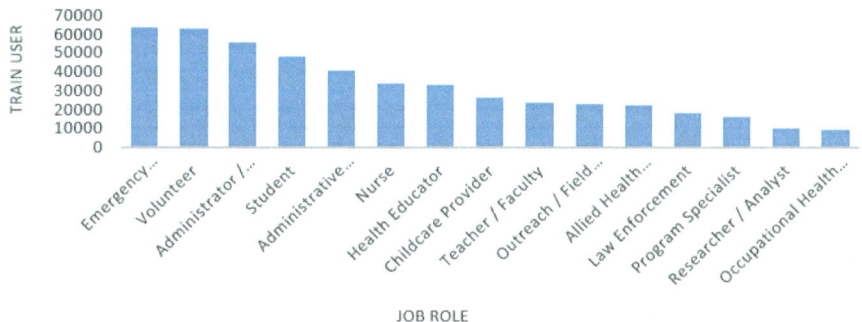

FIGURE 5-2 Top 15 job roles of TRAIN users in nonprofits, private industry, and other sectors.
SOURCE: Bialek presentation, March 22, 2019.

skateboard parks. Leading topic areas for people outside of public health and health care include HIV/AIDS, preparedness and response, communications tools for health care professionals, and the Health Insurance Portability and Accountability Act (HIPAA). Leading topic areas for public health and health care professionals include preparedness and response, HIPAA, people with disabilities, and civil rights. Bialek noted that the data are available to researchers interested in doing further analysis.

Bialek next described work to provide guidance on the skills and competencies important for practicing population health. Population health competencies were intended to be cross-disciplinary and not address a specific role. In developing the competencies, PHF used a lengthy feedback process involving hospitals, the American Association of Medical Colleges, public health agencies, the Association of State and Territorial Health Officials, the National Association of County and City Health Officials, and broad public input. The process resulted in 57 competencies across 6 domains: community engagement, community health assessment, community health improvement planning and action, health equity and cultural awareness, systems thinking, and organizational planning and management.

As Bialek explained, PHF got involved in developing population health competencies after providing public health competencies to hospital professionals at the Association for Community Health Improvement annual meeting. The foundation also hosted a workshop with 40–45 hospital and health professionals to refine the public health competencies. These competencies were ultimately directed toward people working in community benefit for hospitals and health systems. The foundation held several public comment periods to gather input, learned that interest in the competencies extended beyond people working in community benefit, and decided to revise them to make them broadly applicable to people working toward population health in all settings and disciplines.

Bialek next described some of the competencies in a few key domains. Community engagement competencies included describing the historical and current conditions affecting health in a community and collaborating with organizations to maximize use of community assets and resources. For example, Bialek noted that it is important to understand historical conditions with respect to adverse childhood experiences. Community health assessment competencies included describing factors affecting community health (e.g., inequity, income, education, environment, demographic trends, and legislation) and using informatics and information technology to access, collect, analyze, use, maintain, and disseminate data and information. Bialek explained that these data could include electronic health records and information on who is purchasing what, where. Health equity and cultural awareness competencies included communicating in writing and orally with linguistic and cultural proficiency and ensuring that the diversity of individuals and populations is addressed in policies, programs, and services that affect community health. Bialek noted that there are also competencies related to evaluating the extent to which this happens and considering unintended consequences. Within the category of systems thinking, one competency is explaining ways community development is funded to improve the health of populations at the local level. This involves describing activities of community development financial organizations and strategies for leveraging them as funding sources. The systems thinking competency describes the impact the organization is having on the health of the community.

As Bialek explained, PHF has developed training plans to support workers in developing the population health competencies. These plans are a compilation of some of the best trainings available through TRAIN and address specific topics, such as health equity and social determinants of health that cut across many competencies in various domains related to population health.

In closing, Bialek described next steps for PHF regarding TRAIN and the population health competencies. The foundation is exploring adding these competencies into TRAIN to allow people to search for trainings by competency. TRAIN already includes searchable competencies for public health professionals. The foundation is also exploring developing other training plans, similar to the social determinants of health training plan, for people who are not in public health or health care to help them identify what is most important for them to learn regarding population health. Bialek noted that the foundation is also working to disseminate the competencies through a range of partners and networks, using platforms such as presentations, workshops, webinars, and interest groups. For example, the foundation is part of a social determinants innovation collaborative that involves 40–45 health systems and is working to help participating organizations understand and use the competencies.

Be a Change Leader, Build a Culture of Health[4]

Brian Smedley from the National Collaborative for Health Equity (NCHE) and the Robert Wood Johnson Foundation (RWJF) Culture of Health Leaders Program opened by explaining that his presentation would also describe a program focused on building a community of leaders who are well trained to work across sectors and within their own sector to build a culture of health.

The RWJF Culture of Health Leaders Program is relatively young, recruiting its fourth cohort of leaders as of this workshop, although the first cohort has not yet completed it.[5] Smedley pointed out that RWJF's investment in leadership development has been the largest within the health sector, and the foundation has also recognized the need to reach and train leaders in other sectors. The program was developed a few years ago, when RWJF sunsetted some of its legacy leadership programs. RWJF has four new leadership programs:

1. Health Policy Research Scholars, which supports graduate students committed to conducting research to address policy questions involving underserved populations that face inequities;
2. Interdisciplinary Research Leaders, an innovative program that pairs researchers with community members to form more cohesive teams of collaboration across communities and campuses;
3. Clinical Scholars, an innovative program connecting clinical professionals with community members to address problems; and
4. Culture of Health Leaders Program (the topic of Smedley's presentation).

Smedley explained that NCHE co-leads the Culture of Health Leaders Program with CommonHealth ACTION. Other innovative program partners include the Institute for Alternative Futures, the Center for Creative Leadership, the Leadership Learning Community, the American Planning

---

[4] This section summarizes information presented by Brian Smedley from NCHE and the RWJF Culture of Health Leaders Program. The statements made are not endorsed or verified by the National Academies of Sciences, Engineering, and Medicine.

[5] More information about the Culture of Health Leaders Program is available at https://cultureofhealth-leaders.org (accessed May 10, 2021).

Association (APA), and the Build Healthy Places Network, which connects public health with the community development sector.

The Culture of Health Leaders Program is a 3-year, intensive, advanced leadership development initiative that provides formal leadership training, professional coaching, and peer coaching. It challenges participants to conduct strategic, evidence-based work that changes conditions in organizations and communities. It is grounded in the principles of equity and social justice and focuses on addressing the root causes of inequity in systems and structures.

As Smedley described, the program has selected up to 40 leaders per year for the past 3 years from a range of disciplines and sectors, including arts, education, and policy. For example, one leader is a firefighter from Detroit. Current leaders are geographically diverse and represent nearly all 50 states and the District of Columbia; a future goal is to have leaders from all 50 states and the District of Columbia.

Smedley listed some of the characteristics of leadership program participants. They come to the program with well-developed leadership skills and tremendous expertise but are highly motivated, ready to learn, and planning to accelerate their leadership and engage more deeply with communities to realize the vision of healthy, equitable spaces. Participants embrace complexity and risk taking, strive to increase their influence and network more broadly, and intend to extend their work through these networks. Participants must commit 32–38 hours per month for 3 years.

The program model is based around developing four areas of mastery: environment, relationships, change, and the self. Mastery of environment is being able to understand historical and contemporary political and social challenges. Mastery of relationships is being able to bring out the best in others. Mastery of change is sustaining systemic changes. Mastery of self is having awareness and discipline to exert leadership. Smedley highlighted that the goal of the program is for leaders to be at the nexus of these four areas and able to influence others through their decisions, behaviors, and actions.

Smedley outlined the program progression; in year 1, the focus is on competencies related to self and relationships. Information is provided through in-person training, virtual learning, coursework, assessments, executive coaching, and peer coaching. In year 2, the focus is on mastery of environment and change. Activities include executive coaching, peer coaching, and ongoing assessments with the Center for Creative Leadership. In year 3, leaders begin to implement a strategic initiative in their communities focused on all four areas of mastery.

Smedley pointed out that mastery of self includes self-management, self-regulation, self-insight, and self-development (see Figure 5-3). Mastery of relationships includes the ability to build collaborative relation-

Program Competencies

Mastery of Self	Mastery of Relationships	Mastery of Environment	Mastery of Change
Self-management; Self-insight, Self-development	Building Collaborative Relationships	Acts Systematically	Influencing, Leadership, Power
Handles Disequilibrium	Values Diversity	Getting Information, Making Sense of It; Problem Identification	Change Management
Learns Through Others	Brings out the Best in People	Sound Judgment	Communicates
Interpersonal Savvy	Managing Conflict Negotiation	Demonstrates Vision	Risk Taking; Innovation

CULTURE OF HEALTH LEADERS

FIGURE 5-3 Culture of Health Leaders Program competencies.
SOURCE: Smedley presentation, March 22, 2019.

ships and to bring out the best in people working across lines of difference. Mastery of the environment includes acting and thinking systemically, distilling complex information about complex problems that require sound judgment. Mastery of change includes being able to influence and lead others, communicate, and sustain meaningful change.

NONTRADITIONAL STUDENT TRAINING THROUGH THE BLOOMBERG AMERICAN HEALTH INITIATIVE[6]

Michelle Spencer from the Bloomberg American Health Initiative opened by explaining that her presentation would address training nontraditional students in public health through that initiative. Spencer began with some brief history on the initiative.[7] As she explained, about 3 years ago, the Bloomberg Philanthropies provided a $300 million gift to the Johns Hopkins Bloomberg School of Public Health in honor of the school's centennial. The funds were to address the recent decline in health expec-

---

[6] This section summarizes information presented by Michelle Spencer from the Bloomberg American Health Initiative. The statements made are not endorsed or verified by the National Academies of Sciences, Engineering, and Medicine.

[7] More information about the Bloomberg American Health Initiative is available at https://americanhealth.jhu.edu (accessed May 10, 2021).

tancy in the United States. The Bloomberg American Health Initiative aimed to use the tools of public health—education, research, policy, and action—to address health challenges in five focus areas: (1) addiction and overdose, (2) the environment, (3) obesity and the food system, (4) risks to adolescent health, and (5) violence. Cross-cutting themes included social, economic, and health equity; data and evidence; and policy levers, barriers, and needed changes.

This gift provided for 25 endowed professorships and a fellowship program offering up to 50 full tuition annual scholarships for M.P.H. degree students and 10 for Dr.P.H. degree students. As Spencer described, the fellowship program involved three areas of focus: education, research, and policy. The goal of the program is to have an impact and engage individuals in nontraditional spaces with responsibilities and actions that can inadvertently positively affect health outcomes.

As of the date of the workshop, 37 fellows representing 15 states, the District of Columbia, and 1 territory had initiated the program and 2 had completed it. Approximately 40 percent of the fellows represented local, state, and federal health agencies. Others came from nongovernmental organizations, and many had nontraditional backgrounds (outside of public health). Spencer provided examples of a few fellows' experiences. Alison Miller worked for the North Carolina Office of the Chief Medical Examiner and had seen firsthand the growing number of young people who were dying of overdoses. She applied to the fellowship program wanting to understand what her office could do to support people and communities experiencing substance abuse. Amanda Capitummino worked with Sitkans Against Family Violence, a nonprofit organization in Alaska providing services to victims of domestic violence and sexual assault. She wanted to learn what could be done to address violence in her community. Jennifer Spiller in Grand Rapids worked with the Healthy Home Coalition of West Michigan, focusing on environmental challenges in the home. Spiller was interested in addressing what could be done to support healthy housing for individuals with asthma symptoms due to air quality issues. Ashley Hickson in Houston, Texas, worked with the American Heart Association to address food access in communities and implications for obesity, heart disease, and mortality. Veronica Helms from the Department of Housing and Urban Development (HUD) was focused on adolescent health and wanted to know how HUD's health and housing initiatives intersect with adolescent health and what federal-level policies impacting health she could help to inform. The final example was Haven Wheelock in Portland, Oregon, who worked with a nonprofit organization called Outside In, which ran the first publicly funded needle/syringe exchange program.

Spencer explained that each fellowship program applicant was required to submit an application to the program along with their organization. The program could be completed either part time online or full time in Baltimore. While the School of Public Health has clear academic requirements, courses were also informed by fellows' organizations through bimonthly check-in calls. Organizations identified specific topics that would be useful, including health disparities, suicide prevention, and the opioid crisis, from a problem-solving perspective. Some of these topics were addressed through seminars. Participating organizations identified other training needs, including leadership development, advocacy, media and communications, and program implementation. Organizations providing fellows could also receive funding directly through the program for specific public health projects. For example, the Cherokee Nation was funded to conduct data assessments related to opioid use disorders, and ChangeLab Solutions, Indiana University, Child Justice, and the Fort Lauderdale Police Department wanted to conduct research with program faculty, connect with similar organizations around the country, and receive guidance related to policy change.

After completing the program, fellows were required to commit to going back to their organization and staying for at least 1 year. The intent of the program was for the fellows to educate those organizations about the tools of public health, the importance of achieving public health goals, and how public health can inform their processes.

As Spencer noted, nearly two-thirds (62 percent) of fellows were from nontraditional organizations, and 96 percent were women. The fellows represented diversity in terms of organizational and geographic area (see Figures 5-4 and 5-5). Spencer closed by stating that a goal is to have public health advocates in nontraditional public health spaces across the United States.

Obesity and the Food System	MPH	Part-time	ChangeLab Solutions, Oakland, CA
	MPH	Full-time	Research Triangle Institute, Durham, NC
	MPH	Part-Time	Indiana University, Indianapolis, IN
	MPH	Part-Time	National Farm to School Network, Bozeman, MT
Environmental Challenges	MPH	Full-time	Baltimore Heritage, Baltimore, MD
	MPH	Part-time	Food and Water Watch, Washington, DC
	DrPH	Part-time	Deep South Center for Environmental Justice, New Orleans, LA
	DrPH	Part-time	Earthjustice, New York, NY
Violence	MPH	Part-time	Fort Lauderdale Police Department, Fort Lauderdale, FL
	MPH	Part-time	House of Ruth, Baltimore, MD
	MPH	Part-time	Child Justice, Colesville, MD
	MPH	Part-time	International Chiefs of Police, Alexandria, VA
Risks to Adolescent Health	MPH	Part-time	Saginaw County Youth Protection Council Innerlink, Saginaw, MI
	MPH	Part-time	Maplewood Memorial Library, Maplewood, NJ
	MPH	Part-time	Soccer Without Borders, Baltimore, MD
	DrPH	Part-time	Montefiore School Health Program, New York, NY
Addiction and Overdose	MPH	Part-time	Reframe Health and Justice, Washington, DC
	MPH	Part-time	NY/NJ High Intensity Drug Trafficking Area, NJ
	MPH	Part-time	University of Pennsylvania Health System, PA
	DrPH	Part-time	White House Office of National Drug Control Policy, DC

FIGURE 5-4 Incoming 2019 Bloomberg Fellowship collaborating organizations.
SOURCE: Spencer presentation, March 22, 2019.

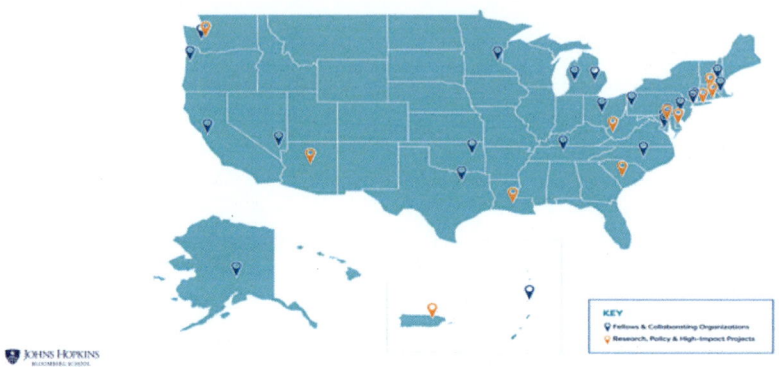

FIGURE 5-5 Geographic footprint of the Bloomberg American Health Initiative.
SOURCE: Spencer presentation, March 22, 2019.

PLANNING AND PUBLIC HEALTH

Sagar Shah spoke on behalf of APA. He described the connection between planning and public health, how APA and the planning community have integrated public health and equity into their activities,[8] and how planning and public health practitioners collaborate in theory and in practice.

Shah began by describing the intersection between planning and public health from a historical perspective. As he explained, until the end of the 19th century, planning and public health were synonymous. By the beginning of the 20th century, public health started moving away from engineering-based solutions to people-based approaches and initiatives, and planners began to focus on designing cities and communities. This changed in the 1980s and 1990s, when public health and planning united with the Healthy Cities movement, which emphasized the importance of addressing social determinants of health. According to Shah, since the beginning of the 21st century, public health and planning have worked together well, but there is still room for improvement.

Many aspects of public health are determined by factors beyond health care. Shah provided several examples of domains for planning healthy communities. One example is whether communities are walk-

---

[8] This section summarizes information presented by Sagar Shah from APA. The statements made are not endorsed or verified by the National Academies of Sciences, Engineering, and Medicine.

able or car dependent, impacting people's ability to be physically active. He noted that subdomains of active living include active transportation (going from one place to another with a purpose) and active recreation (activities such as going to parks and on walks and jogs). Another subdomain of active living is traffic safety. Planners also play an important role in influencing access to healthy foods through land use and zoning decisions and in creating inclusive public spaces that support social cohesion. An additional example was emergency preparedness and climate change. Planning can influence climate change by impacting carbon emissions from automobiles, which vary depending on whether development is sprawled or compact.

Shah next provided background on APA, including its organization and activities related to public health.[9] APA is the largest membership organization for planners in the world, advocating excellence in planning and promoting education and citizen empowerment. Many of its members work in government at various levels. The organization has more than 45,000 members from all states and territories. There are 47 chapters, representing all 50 states, and 21 divisions focused on specific topics or groups of population, including sustainability, transportation, economic development, and women in planning. APA also has interest groups, which are established prior to formal divisions. One such interest group is the Healthy Communities Collaborative; it has more than 750 members, more than half of whom are public health professionals, and is focused on cross-sector collaboration between planning and public health.

APA also has a Planning and Community Health Center, managed by Shah. That center is one of the three flagship sponsored-research programs in APA's research department. The center provides members with tools and training to integrate health and equity into planning at all levels of government. Shah provided some examples of its projects: creating healthy neighborhoods, the role of planners in health impact assessments, benefits of street-scale features, food systems and access to healthy foods, and access to physical activity locations. In recent years, APA's Planning and Community Health Center has also worked to focus on emerging issues, such as the impact of climate change on health and the role of planners, how gentrification impacts health, and how planners can play a role in housing policy. The Center's work falls into three broad categories: (1) applied research, including reviews of the academic and gray literature and development of reports and tools for members; (2) place-based work, including the flagship program PLAN4Health, which provided funding for 35 community coalitions involving public health and planning

---

[9] More information about APA and its initiatives is available at https://www.planning.org (accessed May 10, 2021).

representatives and community-based organizations to address access to healthy foods or access to physical activity locations; and (3) training and education, including webinars, toolkits, and other resources for members. An example is a three-part webinar series on the role of planners in curbing the opioid epidemic.

Shah also provided examples of APA's broader projects. One was a place-based project integrating health and equity into comprehensive plans in collaboration with The Pew Charitable Trusts and RWJF. The partnership has supported three communities in integrating health and equity into their city-level comprehensive plans. Another project involves creating educational models to help planners identify sites for Early Care and Education facilities in areas affected by disasters, accomplished in partnership with the National Environmental Health Association and the Centers for Disease Control and Prevention. Shah noted that partnerships—and particularly cross-sector partnerships—are an important component of APA's strategy. Partners include national membership organizations, federal agencies, foundations, universities, and local organizations.

Shah closed by sharing a joint call to action to promote healthy communities of eight national organizations working at the intersection of built environment and health, including APA, the American Institute of Architects, the American Public Health Association, the American Society of Civil Engineers, the American Society of Landscape Architects, the National Recreation and Park Association, the Urban Land Institute, and the Green Building Council.[10] The goal is to have these organizations' local members come together in their own communities to talk about health and cross-sector partnership.

HEALTH IN ALL POLICIES IN FAIRFAX COUNTY, VIRGINIA[11]

Anna Ricklin from the Fairfax County Health Department in Fairfax County, Virginia, described her role as a "health in all policies manager" and how it helps to promote health in all policies within the department. As Ricklin explained, she has training in public health with urban planning and transportation, having worked previously with APA and the Baltimore City Department of Transportation. Her position is in the Office of Innovation in the Fairfax County Health Department, the goal of which is to promote "Public Health 3.0" and create a culture of health. The

---

[10] For more information, see https://www.planning.org/nationalcenters/health/callto action (accessed May 10, 2021).

[11] This section summarizes information presented by Anna Ricklin from the Fairfax County Health Department in Fairfax County, Virginia. The statements made are not endorsed or verified by the National Academies of Sciences, Engineering, and Medicine.

Office of Innovation also includes a workforce strategist and a research analyst focused on special projects. One of these special projects involved developing a plan to address the opioid crisis within the county. Following delivery of that plan, the county executive hired an opioid director to implement it. The workforce strategist is focused on addressing workforce capacity within the health department, including how best to retain staff and provide career plans and opportunities for growth and development, which may include working with other agencies within Fairfax County and returning to the health department with new knowledge and cross-sector training and experience. Ricklin's role is to serve as an ambassador for public health to agencies across the county, including those not typically considered to be public health actors. She has begun to build relationships with leaders in the departments of planning and zoning, transportation, housing, and neighborhood and community services. She highlighted that having someone from the health department embedded within other agencies has been key to advancing cross-sector collaboration and bringing health into new conversations.

Ricklin described the process to establish her position, noting that before she was even hired, there was an effort to build support for her position with other agencies. For example, during the interview process, Ricklin met with leaders of the county agencies overseeing health, transportation, urban planning, and land development. She noted that the director of the health department wanted these cross-sector leaders to have buy-in on who was hired to ensure that their staff in other departments would know their leadership supported working with the person in Ricklin's position. She said there was initially pushback on hiring a city planner from the human resources department within the health department, because they had never done that before.

To facilitate interaction with staff within the county's land development and zoning agencies, Ricklin's physical office is located in the same building as the Departments of Planning and Zoning and Land Development Services, rather than the health department. Ricklin noted that a key component of her role is "gathering intelligence" through participating in meetings where the health department historically has not been represented, seeking to obtain information about other agencies' plans and priorities and where there might be an opportunity for the health department to engage. For example, the health department could conduct a health impact assessment of a proposed development project. Ricklin completed a "desktop health impact assessment" of a large hospital development where there were concerns about community safety due to increased traffic and other impacts. She used a health equity and social determinants of health lens to assess factors extending beyond increased access to quality health care. Ricklin pointed out that her job is unique, with only "a handful" of health department staff across the country focused on health in all policies as their main job. As she stated, the position provides a new approach to cross-sector partnership and policy making.

Ricklin also described cross-sector training in the county. She noted that a 6-week course, called the Joint Training Academy, was developed out of an initiative called Fairfax First, which was designed to streamline land development. The course is open to all county staff and focuses on the land development process, including the comprehensive plan, zoning, permitting, and other complexities. There is also an ongoing lunch and learn series, for which she presented a session on health and all policies to land development staff. Another example was a healthy community design summit that the health department hosted a few years before with stakeholders from across the county, including leadership from land development, transportation, planning, zoning, and communities.

The county sponsors a Master of Public Administration (M.P.A.) degree at George Mason University for county employees. Students apply through the county, with their supervisor's approval, and take courses in the evenings. The health department also recently finalized a new program for employees to receive a public health certificate at George Mason University that is also paid for by the county. As Ricklin explained, the certificate requires half the credits of an M.P.H. degree, providing an incentive for health department employees to continue their education toward an M.P.H. on their own. She noted that there is interest among health departments in other Northern Virginia cities and counties in offering a similar program to their employees.

DISCUSSION

Gunderson began the discussion portion of the session by encouraging the panelists to ask questions of each other. Ricklin began by asking Spencer how the Bloomberg American Health Initiative has changed the dialogue within the Johns Hopkins Bloomberg School of Public Health about what is public health. Spencer responded that one concrete impact of the initiative has been to demonstrate the need for more flexibility regarding the admission requirements of the School of Public Health. She noted that all fellowship program participants must first apply to the school, which used to recommend that all applicants have at least 2 years of health-related experience. However, lawyers or law enforcement officials who lack this experience would otherwise be good candidates for the program. The school has allowed flexibility in considering the other credentials and experience that these candidates bring and sometimes helped them take classes to qualify for acceptance. She also noted that the leadership of the school and department heads has also recognized the importance of creating courses to meet partner organizations' needs and doing things differently than they have in the past.

After Gunderson opened the discussion to the audience, Donna Grande from the American College of Preventive Medicine pointed out that there are more than 4,000 preventive medicine physicians and residents in medical colleges and schools of public health across the country, who could serve as allies and leaders in promoting community-based change. Grande clarified that preventive medicine physicians are doctors who typically also have an M.P.H. degree and additional training or experience in health departments. She pointed out that they hold about three-quarters of health officer positions. Grande asked Shah for any examples of situations in which APA worked with preventive medicine physicians within health departments or outside of government. While Shah did not have any specific examples to offer, he stated that the eight organizations that formed the call to action he described have been meeting regularly to discuss joint strategy and long-term goals. He noted that there has been discussion about including other organizations in the call to action, such as a transportation organization, and there could potentially be an opportunity to include preventive medicine physicians as well.

Both Gunderson and Kevin Barnett from the Public Health Institute and the California Health Workforce Alliance used the terms "disruptors" and "transformational" to describe the panelists. To achieve similar transformational, structural change in other organizations, Gunderson asked whether there is a need for more individual disruptors or if additional, broader changes must take place within organizations or government agencies. Bialek responded that, in collaboration with the Center for Creative Leadership and Leadership Learning Community, they are building "collaborative leadership," which they define as leadership that understands the need for broader frames and ways of communicating across fields of understanding and deep engagement with communities. Bialek pointed out that common characteristics of many of RWJF's leadership programs are that community linkages are critically important and community members have power. He stated that he believes public health is moving toward building collective efficacy and harnessing political power, clarifying that if the ultimate goal is to build collective power, collaborative leadership is essential.

Hanh Cao Yu from The California Endowment added that she appreciated Wiggins's comment that CHW training often involves popular education. She noted that her organization is focused on power building involving those most affected, which resonates with the community rootedness and attention to well-being of the CHW role. Yu also highlighted an important question raised by Barnett of how to ensure that health care providers return to their communities following formal education and training.

Michael Rhein from the Institute for Public Health Innovation asked Ricklin whether she received pushback from other agencies that the health in all policies concept is too centered on public health and would be better if it were more broadly focused on equitable, prosperous communities. Ricklin responded that while the terminology "health in all policies" may not always resonate across agencies, the concepts do, and she often explains the concepts using examples. She noted that she is still working on developing the best messaging but generally recommends using other agencies' language and terminology whenever possible. Ricklin added that the concept of equity has gained momentum in the county, such as the One Fairfax policy adopted in 2017 that requires using an equity lens with all policy-making projects across the county. Ricklin is part of a team led by the chief equity officer to operationalize that policy. Points made by the speakers in this section are highlighted below (see Box 5-1).

BOX 5-1
Points Made by Individual Speakers and Participants

- Workers both within and outside of public health are seeking training on a range of topics related to population health, including use of data, healthy homes, food insecurity, and building construction principles. (Bialek)
- The Robert Wood Johnson Foundation's Culture of Health Leaders Program is focused on four key areas of mastery: environment, relationships, change, and self. (Smedley)
- The success of the Bloomberg American Health Initiative has pointed to the need for flexibility in considering the full range of credentials and experience that candidates bring, even when they lack formal public health experience. (Spencer)
- Planners can play an important role in influencing aspects of public health, including walkable neighborhoods, access to healthy foods, inclusive public spaces, emergency preparedness, and climate change. (Shah)
- Having someone from the health department embedded within other agencies is key to advancing cross-sector collaboration and bringing health into new conversations. (Ricklin)

NOTE: This list is the rapporteurs' summary of the main points made by individual speakers and participants (noted in parentheses) and does not reflect any consensus among workshop participants or endorsement by the National Academies of Sciences, Engineering, and Medicine.

6

Breakout Session: Moving Toward a Population Health Workforce Exercise[1]

INSTRUCTIONS

Workshop participants were invited to participate in an interactive exercise related to the population health workforce. The activity involved considering workforce development in the context of larger strategies related to social determinants of health. Marthe Gold from The New York Academy of Medicine facilitated the exercise; the in-person participants were assigned a topic of school absenteeism, food security, or affordable housing and divided into groups of five to six people. A brief case study was provided for each topic. Each group was instructed to identify a facilitator to manage the conversation and a scribe to write down key points of discussion. Next, the activity required that each group identify an "honest broker" who would be likely to convene a group in the community on the selected topic. One group member would play the role of the convener, and other group members were asked to take on the roles of other community stakeholders who would be interested in addressing the issue.

Gold asked participants to consider the strategies and tactics related to training and workforce development that could be used to address the issue provided and to identify potential stakeholders and payers. Participants were specifically directed to consider potential funding sources for

---

[1] This section describes the discussions that occurred during the breakout session. Statements, recommendations, and opinions expressed are those of individual participants and should not be construed as reflecting any group consensus.

the recommended strategies and tactics, including whether new funds would be needed or if a cross-sector partner would provide funding. Each group was asked to complete a worksheet identifying the issue, convener, partners, potential strategies, and tactics. Appendix D presents the instructions for the small group exercise, the three scenarios, and the worksheet.

Gold shared a conceptual model describing pathways to health equity (see Figure 6-1) that was published in a prior National Academies report (NASEM, 2017). She noted that a goal of the exercise was to consider how to use workforce strategies to promote equity within communities, as described in the model. Gold also referenced Figure 1-1, demonstrating that training runs along a continuum from formal and structured to informal and unstructured. That figure provides examples of types of training at multiple points along the continuum.

DISCUSSION

After 40 minutes of small group discussion, the workshop participants reconvened to share key takeaways from each group's conversation. A representative from one of two groups focused on school absenteeism spoke first. As was explained, the scenario involved a school with a high rate of chronic absenteeism. The group identified the school to be the reluctant convener, but not the funder, as schools already have a

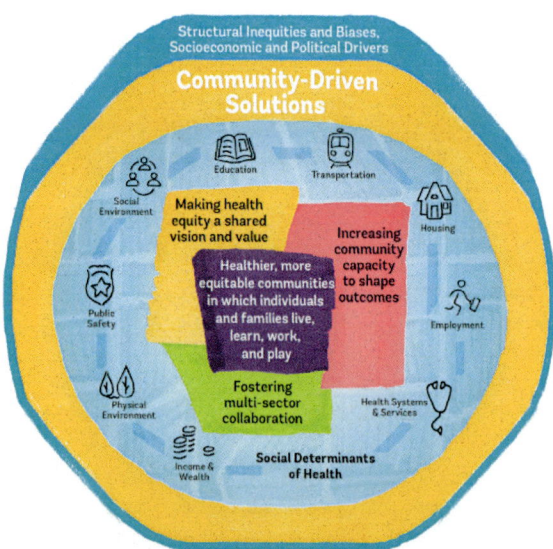

FIGURE 6-1 Conceptual model describing Pathways to Health Equity.
SOURCES: Gold presentation, March 22, 2019; NASEM, 2017.

lot of responsibilities. Additional partners identified include employers, banks, legislators, school resource officers, student attendance support staff, public housing providers, school athletics, and local government. The group focused on upstream factors and recommended a multigenerational approach involving parents and caregivers as well as students, noting that if caregivers feel supported, they are more likely to be able to support the children. Specific strategies identified based on the experience of group members included having a community bank invest in a pilot in one school and work to get other businesses involved, having the school convene the partners previously identified to discuss the problem and identify solutions, and holding focus groups to learn from the community regarding levers that could address the underlying causes of absenteeism. An additional strategy was to have the county executive declare school absenteeism a priority. In response to a question from Gold regarding how the group specifically addressed training needs, it was noted that there was discussion about training for school staff on absenteeism, and they determined that training for existing staff would likely be more effective than hiring new staff.

A second group addressing school absenteeism was led by Lisa Kaplowitz, a physician in a job transition who was returning to local public health. Kaplowitz explained that her group spent time discussing the reasons for absenteeism, including violence, homelessness, and health issues, and how each of these reasons could bring additional partners to the table, including law enforcement, homeless shelters, school nurses, health care providers, and parents. The group pointed to the need to improve communication among the diverse group of partners and suggested that community health workers (CHWs) could play a role in educating diverse stakeholders about the issues, potential solutions, and partners who would be most trusted in delivering them. It was also suggested that absenteeism could present a workforce issue for major employers in the area if it was keeping parents at home. Additional support and funding could come from the major employers and the hospital, which could use community benefit funds to address the problem.

The representative from the group focused on affordable housing explained that their scenario involved a community with high rates of displacement and residents who are rent burdened, creating a need to address affordable housing. Partners identified included the local government housing authority, health care institutions, philanthropy, state-based organizations, community-oriented organizations, advocacy groups, faith-based community representatives, and academic experts. The group selected a local philanthropic group to serve as the neutral convener, as this group could likely address the interests of the people at risk. One workforce-specific strategy that the group discussed was training for housing authority and hospital staff on how to bring a social determinants lens to their work. It was also noted that the high cost of housing could be a workforce issue for the health care system because there is often poor job satisfaction and high turnover when health care employees cannot afford to live near their workplace. Another strategy was to fund an epidemiologist to provide information to the housing authority on the connection between social determinants of health and health outcomes.

Michael Rhein from the Institute for Public Health Innovation (IPHI) reported for the group focused on food insecurity, explaining that his group's scenario involved a town experiencing food insecurity issues that was interested in developing a comprehensive plan to address the issue. He likened this scenario to IPHI's work involving a public health entity as the convener of a nonincorporated multi-sectoral coalition, which the group termed the Food Equity Council. One strategy the group suggested was to work with school administrators to adopt the community eligibility provisions of Title I. The group recommended providing advocacy training for parents, teachers, and community members along with issue training for the public health community, school community groups, and school administrators on the importance of addressing food insecurity and potential actions. Following the adoption of any policy change, the group recommended additional training on policy implementation and a communications campaign for educators and school staff. An additional strategy was to lead a campaign to bring a full-service grocery store back to the neighborhood; the scenario noted that one had recently closed. Workforces involved with this strategy could include traditional governmental public health planners, the economic development sector, and community members. Tactics involved advocacy training and workforce development training for CHWs, who could lead the advocacy campaign for the store in collaboration with other community residents. There was also a suggestion that the public health sector receive training on economic development and potential financing mechanisms for the new store and that the economic development sector receive training on the role of food access in ensuring healthy and prosperous communities.

In closing, Gold acknowledged that while it may have been difficult for workshop participants to identify numerous workforce or training strategies in the limited time for the exercise, the activity helped them consider the information presented at the workshop.

7

Reflections on the Day and Closing Remarks

Joshua Sharfstein from the Johns Hopkins Bloomberg School of Public Health concluded the day by reflecting on the reasons for the workshop and key takeaways. Sharfstein noted that one reason was the importance of considering who is responsible for addressing the many factors related to population health. The planning committee decided to focus on training for public health and medical professionals, community health workers (CHWs), and other sectors in a single workshop because these three workforces are all important for promoting population health.

Sharfstein highlighted some opportunities and challenges presented in each panel. In the first panel, Perspectives from Professional and Accrediting Organizations, he sees as an opportunity the fact that some people in public health aspire to be effective population health leaders. Challenges include large training gaps and the lack of a direct connection between the current public health and health care education and accreditation system and population health needs. With respect to the second panel, The Community Health Workforce, Sharfstein highlighted as opportunities the enthusiasm of CHWs, their combination of lived experience plus additional training, and the examples of how they can make a significant difference in people's lives. He noted that challenges include that CHWs are often not well employed and not incentivized to be leveraged by the health care system, which limits training and professional development opportunities. He sees a particularly promising model in Maryland; it involves using millions of dollars from the health care system to train and hire many CHWs. With respect to the third panel, Cross-Sector Workforce:

National and Local Examples, Sharfstein shared that a key takeaway is the potential interest among other sectors in receiving training on and further engaging with public health. He noted that a limitation in making public health training relevant to other sectors could be the language, or framing, that is used. He also noted that there may not be many job opportunities available for a public health–trained planner or transportation official.

Sharfstein stated that he supported addressing the three workforce issues in a single meeting in order to demonstrate how the three workforces could come together to address problems. He suggested that a future need is for foundations, governments, and others to invest in the workforce at the juncture between public health, health care, CHWs, and other sectors. One way to do so could be to bring these three areas of training together in an interprofessional conference that allows workers from multiple disciplines to jointly receive training on how to work together to achieve specific goals. In regard to the small group exercise, Sharfstein explained that he also expects that a political priority—such as school absenteeism, affordable housing, or food insecurity—could provide an opportunity for increased investment in the workforce across all three areas discussed during the workshop.

Finally, Sharfstein offered an opportunity for workshop participants to offer their own reflections and concluding remarks. Lourdes Rodriguez from the Center for Place-Based Initiatives at the Dell Medical School at The University of Texas at Austin suggested that if public health recommends a "health in all policies approach," in which other disciplines apply public health principles to their work, public health could similarly learn from other sectors that have mastered other skills, such as logistics, communications, customer satisfaction, and engineering, and apply these principles to public health work. Rodriguez also highlighted some key issues for future consideration related to CHWs, including the science to support their use, sustainable funding strategies, and the importance of training not just them but also the "ecosystem" in which they work. She also noted the importance of cross-sector funding for initiatives that bring a broad range of stakeholders together.

Cathy Baase from the Michigan Health Improvement Alliance added that, in addition to workforce training needs, an enabling framework of multi-stakeholder collaboratives and partnerships is important in addressing the issues discussed. She noted that "integrator organizations" could be useful in pulling together multi-stakeholder collaboratives at the community level. This type of entity could be jointly funded by multiple stakeholders and provide a vehicle to bring together public health, health care, businesses, community-based organizations, and other partners. In response to a question from Sharfstein about what could be done to strengthen these entities from a workforce training perspective, Baase stated that she is not aware of any training or credentialing specific for multi-sectoral entities, as each sector typically provides its own training, but it could be something to consider for the future.

Noelle Wiggins from the Oregon Community Health Workers Association highlighted a few takeaways regarding strategies for fully integrating CHWs in population health work. She noted that it is important to recognize CHWs as a discrete and uniquely important group of individuals and pointed to the value of the CHW model as providing more than navigation to health services. As the profession is rooted in political and social justice organizing within communities, Wiggins suggested that with community organizing training, CHWs may be able to play the role of community organizer to address pressing issues, such as a housing crisis.

Marthe Gold from The New York Academy of Medicine suggested an option could be to change the term "CHW" to "community worker," as the role may reach beyond health and health care. She noted that this revised terminology may make it easier to obtain funding for community workers from entities focused on improving quality of life and well-being in communities.

Terry Allan from the Cuyahoga County Health Department in Greater Cleveland highlighted Figure 3-3 from Kalpana Ramiah's presentation demonstrating the spectrum of community-integrated care using food security as an example. It noted that there are upstream and downstream strategies for addressing the issue involving individual patients and the community at large. Just as multiple strategies may be needed to address food insecurity, the workshop demonstrated that multiple workforces may also be needed.

Sanne Magnan from the University of Minnesota noted that a key question stemming from the public health panel is whether the right people are being targeted for the right training and professional development opportunities. Another important question, she noted, is how to keep equity at the forefront of population health work. She also addressed Shreya Kangovi's analogy of whether the goal with population health workforce development is to train firefighters or put out fires. While Kangovi had recommended that the focus be on the end goal of putting out fires, Magnan suggested that it is important to both maintain focus on the end goal and train workers to be good at their jobs. She pointed out that without training, the firefighters—or other workers—would likely become overwhelmed. She also suggested that more training is needed to prevent fires from being started (prevent the problem from arising in the first place).

Regarding the cross-sector panel, Magnan noted that she appreciated that Anna Ricklin from the Fairfax County Health Department was embedded within the zoning and community development office. She suggested that it is important for the health sector to "learn the language" of other sectors, noting that the reverse (trying to force health in all policies) could be perceived as arrogant. One option could be to develop common framing and terminology that is used across sectors. Magnan also acknowledged that while the meeting called for systemic changes to support population health, change is difficult, and it initially may not be easy to accept new ways of doing things or new partners. Points made by the speakers in this section are highlighted below (see Box 7-1).

BOX 7-1
Points Made by Individual Speakers and Participants

- Key challenges for the public health workforce include large training gaps and the lack of direct connection between the current public health and health care education and accreditation system, and population health needs. (Sharfstein)
- Community health workers are often not well used and not incentivized to be used through the health care system, limiting their training and professional development opportunities. (Sharfstein)
- A limitation in making public health training and principles relevant to other sectors could be the terminology or framing that is used. (Gold, Magnan, Sharfstein)
- While public health advocates a "health in all policies" approach, the discipline could similarly learn from other sectors that have mastered other skills and principles and apply them to public health work. (Magnan, Rodriguez)

NOTE: This list is the rapporteurs' summary of the main points made by individual speakers and participants (noted in parentheses) and does not reflect any consensus among workshop participants or endorsement by the National Academies of Sciences, Engineering, and Medicine.

Appendix A

References

AEH (America's Essential Hospitals). 2016. *Essential hospitals population health survey.* https://essentialhospitals.org/institute/institutepopulation-health-at-essential-hospitals-a-road-map-to-community-integrated-health-care (accessed May 10, 2021).

ASPPH (Association of Schools & Programs of Public Health). 2015. *Population health across all professions.* https://www.aspph.org/ftf-reports/population-health-in-all-professions (accessed May 10, 2021).

California Future Health Workforce Commission. 2019. *Meeting the demand for health: Final report of the California Future Health Workforce Commission.* https://futurehealthworkforce.org/wp-content/uploads/2019/03/MeetingDemandForHealthFinalReportCFHWC.pdf (accessed May 10, 2021).

CMS (Centers for Medicare & Medicaid Services). 2016. *Mapping Medicare disparities.* http://data.cms.gov/mapping-medicare-disparities (accessed May 10, 2021).

Hester, J. A., J. Auerbach, D. I. Chang, S. Magnan, and J. Monroe. 2015. *Opportunity knocks again for population health: Round two in state innovation models.* NAM Perspectives. Discussion Paper, National Academy of Medicine, Washington, DC. https://doi.org/10.31478/201504i.

IOM (Institute of Medicine). 2004. *In the nation's compelling interest: Ensuring diversity in the health-care workforce.* Washington, DC: The National Academies Press. https://doi.org/10.17226/10885.

IOM and NRC (National Research Council). 2015. *Transforming the workforce for children birth through age 8: A unifying foundation.* Washington, DC: The National Academies Press. https://doi.org/10.17226/19401.

Kangovi, S., N. Mitra, D. Grande, M. L. White, S. McCollum, J. Sellman, R. P. Shannon, and J. A. Long. 2014. Patient-centered community health worker intervention to improve posthospital outcomes: A randomized clinical trial. *JAMA Internal Medicine* 174(4):535–543.

Kangovi, S., N. Mitra, D. Grande, H. Huo, R. A. Smith, and J. A. Long. 2017. Community health worker support for disadvantaged patients with multiple chronic diseases: A randomized clinical trial. *American Journal of Public Health* 107(10):1660–1667.

NASEM (National Academies of Sciences, Engineering, and Medicine). 2017. *Communities in action: Pathways to health equity.* Washington, DC: The National Academies Press. https://doi.org/10.17226/24624.

NASEM. 2019a. *Integrating social care into the delivery of health care: Moving upstream to improve the nation's health.* Washington, DC: The National Academies Press. https://doi.org/10.17226/25467.

NASEM. 2019b. *Vibrant and healthy kids: Aligning science, practice, and policy to advance health equity.* Washington, DC: The National Academies Press. https://doi.org/10.17226/25466.

Nkonki, L., J. Cliff, and D. Sanders. 2011. Lay health worker attrition: Important but often ignored. *Bulletin of the World Health Organization* 89:919–923.

PCHI (Pathways Community HUB Institute). 2019. *Pathways Community HUB Model overview.* https://pchi-hub.com (accessed May 10, 2021).

PH WINS (Public Health Workforce Interests and Needs Survey). 2019. *Journal of Public Health Management and Practice* 25(S2). https://journals.lww.com/jphmp/toc/2019/03001 (accessed May 10, 2021).

Roberson, B., and K. Ramiah. 2018. *Essential data: Our hospitals, our patients.* Washington, DC: America's Essential Hospitals.

Appendix B

Workshop Agenda

Thursday, March 21, 2019

Keck Center Room 100
500 Fifth Street, NW
Washington, DC 20001

8:00 am	**Welcome and Introduction** Sanne Magnan, Roundtable Co-Chair, *University of Minnesota*
8:10 am	**Keynote and Q&A** Moderator: Sanne Magnan Presenter: Kevin Barnett, *Public Health Institute and the California Health Workforce Alliance*
8:45 am	**Panel 1: Perspectives from Professional and Accrediting Organizations** Moderator: Phyllis Meadows, *The Kresge Foundation* Presenters: Brian Castrucci, *de Beaumont Foundation* Kalpana Ramiah, *America's Essential Hospitals*

Discussants:
Laura Rasar King, *Council on Education for Public Health*
Kaye Bender, *Public Health Accreditation Board*
Lisa Howley, *Association of American Medical Colleges*

9:40 am **Discussion and Q&A**
Moderator: Phyllis Meadows

10:00 am **Break**

10:10 am **Panel 2: The Community Health Workforce**
Moderator: Karen Murphy, *Geisinger*

Presenters:
Community Health Worker Panel:
Shanteny Jackson, *Richmond City Health District and Virginia Community Health Worker Association*
Kevin Jordan, *Damien Ministries and Maryland Community Health Worker Advisory Committee*
Orson Brown, *Penn Center for Community Health Workers*
Adriana Rodriguez Palacios, *Oregon Community Health Worker Association*
Shreya Kangovi, *Penn Center for Community Health Workers*
Noelle Wiggins, *Oregon Community Health Workers Association*
Michael Rhein and Dwyan Monroe, *Institute for Public Health Innovation*
Katie Wunderlich, *Maryland Health Services Cost Review Commission*

11:15 am **Discussion and Q&A**
Moderator: Karen Murphy

11:30 am **Lunch Break**

12:30 pm **Panel 3: Cross-Sector Workforce: National and Local Examples**
Moderator: Gary Gunderson, *Wake Forest Baptist Medical Center and Stakeholder Health*

APPENDIX B 75

                Presenters:
                Ron Bialek, *Public Health Foundation*
                Brian Smedley, *National Collaborative for Health Equity* and
                    Robert Wood Johnson Foundation Culture of Health Leaders
                Michelle Spencer, *Johns Hopkins Bloomberg School of Public*
                    Health and *Bloomberg American Health Initiative*
                Sagar Shah, *American Planning Association*
                Anna Ricklin, *Fairfax County Health Department*

1:40 pm   **Discussion and Q&A**
                Moderator: Gary Gunderson

1:55 pm   **Group Exercise and Reporting Back**
                Moderator: Marthe Gold, *The New York Academy of Medicine*

3:00 pm   **Reflections on the Day and Closing Remarks**
                Joshua Sharfstein, Roundtable Co-Chair, *Johns Hopkins*
                    Bloomberg School of Public Health

3:30 pm   **Adjourn**

Appendix C

Biosketches of Speakers, Moderators, and Planning Committee Members[1]

Kevin Barnett,* Dr.P.H., M.A., is a senior investigator at the Public Health Institute, where he has led research and fieldwork in hospital community benefit and health workforce diversity for more than two decades, working with hospitals, government agencies, and community stakeholders across the country.

Recent work includes a study of community health assessments and implementation strategies for the Centers for Disease Control and Prevention and a national initiative funded by The Kresge Foundation to align and focus investments by hospitals, other health-sector stakeholders, and financial institutions in low-income communities.

Current work includes a partnership with the Governance Institute and Stakeholder Health with funding from the Robert Wood Johnson Foundation to build place-based population health knowledge among hospital board members and senior leadership, a national study of hospital interventions to address food insecurity, and a partnership with the Carsey School of Public Policy to convene regional meetings of hospital and community teams with community development financial institutions to design intersectoral health improvement strategies. He serves as the co-director of the California Health Workforce Alliance and is on the boards of directors of Communities Joined in Action and Trinity Health System.

---

[1] * Denotes planning committee member; † denotes roundtable member.

Kaye Bender, Ph.D., RN, FAAN, has been the president and the chief executive officer of the Public Health Accreditation Board (PHAB) since 2009. Before that, she worked in local public health for several years in Mississippi and was the deputy state health officer for the Mississippi Department of Health for 12 years. She was also the dean of the University of Mississippi Medical Center for 6 years. She chaired the Exploring Accreditation Steering Committee, the precursor study for the establishment of PHAB. Dr. Bender has served on several Institute of Medicine study committees related to public health and nursing. She is an active member of the American Public Health Association and a fellow in the American Academy of Nursing. She is also a board member of the National Board of Public Health Examiners. She has numerous publications and presentations related to governmental public health infrastructure improvement.

Ron Bialek, M.P.P., took over as the executive director of the Public Health Foundation (PHF) in 1996, with 15 years of experience in public health practice and in academia, and became the president of PHF in June 1999. He brings to PHF a wealth of experience in state and local public health practice and linking public health practitioners with academic institutions. Mr. Bialek manages all aspects of the organization and is responsible for the quality of its products. He directed PHF activities over the past 3 years that have led to using distance learning techniques to train more than 10,000 public health professionals annually. Mr. Bialek serves on a variety of government advisory groups and co-chaired the Managed Care and Public Health subcommittee of the Public Health Functions Working Group. He works closely with the PHF board of directors and public health professionals to develop and implement research, training, and technical assistance activities to benefit public health agencies in their performance of public health services.

Before joining PHF, Mr. Bialek was on the faculty of the Johns Hopkins Bloomberg School of Public Health for 9 years and served as the director of the Johns Hopkins Health Program Alliance. In both roles, Mr. Bialek took the theory of public health practice out into the field and developed an outstanding reputation locally and nationally for his efforts in facilitating linkages between academic institutions and public health agencies. At the national level, he has directed such projects as the Public Health Faculty/Agency Forum and the Council on Linkages Between Academia and Public Health Practice. The forum project resulted in recommendations for improving the relevance of public health education to practice and spelled out the various competencies that are desirable for practicing public health. Mr. Bialek still serves as the director of the Council on Linkages and continues to play a key role in developing strategies and programs to implement the forum recommendations throughout the country. In addition, Mr. Bialek is co-directing a national effort to develop public health practice guidelines for use by public and private organizations with population-based responsibilities.

At the state and local levels, Mr. Bialek has done much to improve collaboration between public health agencies and Johns Hopkins. He developed and directed projects that included assessing community public health needs and resources, creating evaluation protocols for local health department services, providing technical support to and staffing for the Maryland Association of County Health Officers, and establishing a public health grand rounds series for state and local health department employees. Mr. Bialek co-chaired the Coalition for Local Public Health in Maryland, which was successful in getting signed into law certain funding mandates to support essential local public health services. He has also served on several state committees and is currently a member of the Prevention Block Grant Advisory Committee for the Maryland Department of Health and Mental Hygiene.

Mr. Bialek also has extensive teaching experience in the areas of public health practice, AIDS health policy and management, and community health assessment. He has provided community health assessment training to more than 200 health departments and community-based organizations, and he is currently developing a distance learning course in this topic area for the Centers for Disease Control and Prevention. Mr. Bialek received his B.A. in political science and M.P.P. in public policy from Johns Hopkins University.

Nisha Botchwey, Ph.D.,* is an associate professor of city and regional planning at the Georgia Institute of Technology and an adjunct professor in the Emory University School of Public Health. An expert in health and the built environment as well as community engagement, she holds graduate degrees in both urban planning and public health. Dr. Botchwey co-directs the National Physical Activity Research Center and both the Atlanta Neighborhood Quality of Life and Health Dashboard and the data dashboard for Health, Environment, and Livability for Fulton County. She also directs the Built Environment and Public Health Clearinghouse.

Dr. Botchwey's research focuses on health and the built environment, health equity, community engagement, and data dashboards for evidence-based planning and practice. She is the co-author of *Health Impact Assessment in the USA* (2014), the convener of a national expert panel on interdisciplinary workforce training between the public health and community design fields, and the author of numerous articles, scientific presentations, and workshops. Dr. Botchwey has won distinctions, including a National Science Foundation ADVANCE Woman of Excellence Faculty Award, a Hesburgh Award Teaching Fellowship from Georgia Tech, the Georgia Power Professor of Excellence Award, a Rockefeller-Penn Fellowship from the University of Pennsylvania School of Nursing, and a Nominated Changemaker by the Obama White House Council on Women and Girls. She has also served on the advisory committee to the director for Centers for Disease Control and Prevention and is a member of the Social Sciences Panel for the Ford Foundation's Fellowship Program and the Voices for Healthy Kids Strategic Advisory Committee for the American Heart Association.

Orson Brown, CHW, is a senior community health worker (CHW) at the Penn Center for Community Health Workers, a national center of excellence dedicated to advancing health in low-income populations through effective CHW programs. Mr. Brown has provided intensive, personalized support to hundreds of patients to help them set and achieve health goals. In addition to his direct work with patients, he has trained new CHWs across the country and taught medical students about the social determinants of health. Mr. Brown also mentors youth who live in Southwest Philadelphia and serves as a deacon in his church.

Brian C. Castrucci, Dr.P.H., M.A., is the chief executive officer at the de Beaumont Foundation. In just 6 years, he has built the foundation into a leading voice in health philanthropy and public health practice. As an award-winning epidemiologist with 10 years of experience working in state and local health departments, Dr. Castrucci brings a unique perspective to the philanthropic sector that allows him to shape and implement visionary and practical initiatives and partnerships and bring together research and practice to improve public health.

Under his leadership, the de Beaumont Foundation is advancing policy, building partnerships, and strengthening the public health system to create communities where people can achieve their best possible health. The projects he has spearheaded include CityHealth, the BUILD Health Challenge, and the Public Health Workforce Interests and Needs Survey.

Dr. Castrucci has published more than 50 articles in the areas of public health systems and services research, maternal and child health, health promotion, and chronic disease prevention. His recent work has focused on the public health needs of large cities, the need for better data systems, and public health system improvements. He is also an editor and a contributing author to *The Practical Playbook: Public Health and Primary Care Together*, published by Oxford University Press in 2015.

Dr. Castrucci earned his Dr.P.H. at the University of North Carolina at Chapel Hill Gillings School of Global Public Health. He graduated summa cum laude with a B.A. in political science from North Carolina State University and an M.A. in sociomedical sciences from Columbia University.

Marthe Gold, M.D., M.P.H.,† joined The New York Academy of Medicine in 2015 as a senior scholar, where her primary focus is on implementing methods to gain informed public participation in decisions that affect them. Nationally, she has worked in different communities to capture resident guidance for decision makers interested in implementing health-related policy changes to advance the health of the populations they serve. A graduate of the Tufts University School of Medicine and the Columbia University Mailman School of Public Health, Dr. Gold has clinical training in family medicine and practiced in rural and urban underserved communities. From 1990 to 1996, she served as the senior policy advisor in the Office of the Assistant Secretary for Health in the Department of Health and Human Services. She returned to her native New York in 1997 to chair the Department of Community Health and Social Medicine at the City University of New York Medical School, whose mission is to train a diverse student body for primary care practice in underserved New York communities. A member of the National Academy of Medicine, Dr. Gold currently serves on the National Academies of Sciences, Engineering, and Medicine's Roundtable on Population Health. She is a member of the New England Comparative Effectiveness Public Advisory Council and the immediate past president of the International Society for Priorities in Health.

Gary R. Gunderson, Ph.D.,*† was appointed in July 2012 to oversee spiritual care services for patients, families, and medical center staff. He supervises six departments: CareNet Counseling, Chaplaincy and Clinical Ministries (including the Clinical Pastoral Education program), FaithHealth Education, Community Engagement, the Center for Congregational Health, and FaithHealthNC. Dr. Gunderson also nurtures relationships with more than 4,300 Baptist congregations throughout North Carolina and other large networks of the center's patients' faith groups.

A recognized expert in congregations and health, Dr. Gunderson previously served as the senior vice president of the Faith and Health Division of Methodist Le Bonheur Healthcare in Memphis, Tennessee. In his 7 years there, he developed a new model of congregational health that became widely known as the "Memphis Model."

Dr. Gunderson became involved in public health through his work with former President Jimmy Carter in Atlanta; he directed the Interfaith Health Program at the Carter Center for a decade. The Interfaith Health Program moved from the Carter Center to the Emory University Rollins School of Public Health, where Dr. Gunderson became a research assistant professor in international health. He also served as a visiting professor in family medicine and community health at the University of Cape Town, South Africa.

Dr. Gunderson has worked extensively with the White House Office of Faith-Based and Neighborhood Partnerships. He serves as the secretary for Stakeholder Health, a group of 39 health systems committed to more effective engagement with the poor in their communities. He brought the Leading Causes of Life Initiative, an international and interdisciplinary group of fellows working to build an intellectual foundation beyond the purely medical paradigm, to Wake Forest Baptist. He was the lead author for a paper based on this work and published by the National Academy of Medicine titled "The Health of Complex Human Populations."

In addition to his role in Faith and Health Ministries, Dr. Gunderson holds faculty appointments at the Wake Forest School of Divinity and in Public Health Sciences. A Wake Forest University alumnus, Dr. Gunderson has a master of divinity from Emory University in Atlanta, a doctorate of ministry from the Interdenominational Theological Center in Atlanta, and an honorary doctorate of divinity from the Chicago Theological Seminary.

Lisa Howley, Ph.D., is an experienced educational psychologist who has spent more than 20 years in the field of medical education supporting learners and faculty, conducting research, and developing curricula. She joined the Association of American Medical Colleges in 2016 to advance the continuum of medical education, support experiential learning, and drive curricular transformation. Before that, she spent 8 years as the associate designated institutional officer and assistant vice president of Medical Education and Physician Development for the Carolinas Health-Care System in North Carolina. In that role, she led a number of medical education initiatives across the professional development continuum, including graduate medical education accreditation and physician leadership development for the large integrated health care system. She concurrently served as an associate professor at the University of North Carolina (UNC) School of Medicine, where she led curriculum and faculty development. She also held a faculty appointment in educational research at UNC at Charlotte, where she taught social science research methods and led or collaborated on numerous studies of effective education. From 1996 to 2001, she was a member of the medical education faculty at the University of Virginia School of Medicine, where she designed and led performance-based assessments and simulation-enhanced curricula. She received her bachelor's in psychology from the University of Central Florida and both her master of education and Ph.D. in educational psychology from the University of Virginia.

Shanteny Jackson, M.A., is a bilingual certified community health worker in the Richmond City health district. She is also the president of the Virginia Community Health Worker Association. Ms. Jackson holds a master's in counseling with a concentration in human services and addiction. She is known as a compassionate collaborator and community advocate. Ms. Jackson has a long-standing service background, with a diverse set of work experiences. She enjoys giving back and being a helpful resource to her community. In her current role, Ms. Jackson has had the opportunity to lead community and social projects.

Kevin Jordan, CHW, is a community health worker (CHW) currently working with Damien Ministries in overseeing its HIV prevention services in Washington, DC. The scope of his work ranges from street outreach to administrative and data reporting to funders. Mr. Jordan has 5 years of combined experience in public health, particularly in the HIV field.

Mr. Jordan first started as a peer advocate for the Children's National Adolescent Education Program, a high school program for Washington, DC, public school students. He was an intern at the World Bank Group, Sustainable Development Network, where he had the opportunity to provide technical support. He volunteered for La Clinica del Pueblo and shortly after became a Promotor de Salud ("health promoter," or CHW). Mr. Jordan was then appointed to the health impact specialist position at the District of Columbia Department of Health, working on the IMPACT DMV 1509 project, a Centers for Disease Control and Prevention–funded grant that expands pre-exposure prophylaxis coverage and creates a holistic care model for populations at risk in the Washington, DC, metropolitan area.

Mr. Jordan is a member of the University of Maryland, College Park, Community Advisory Board for Deferred Action for Childhood Arrivals (DACA) students. He is also part of the focus group for the research portion of the project as a DACA recipient himself. Additionally, he is a member of the Maryland Community Health Worker Advisory Committee, appointed by Governor Larry Hogan. He is also involved with the Institute for Public Health Innovation Professional Association of Community Health Workers and the District of Columbia Department of Health's CHW committee.

Shreya Kangovi, M.D., M.H.S.P., is the founding executive director of the Penn Center for Community Health Workers, a national center of excellence dedicated to advancing health in low-income populations through effective community health worker (CHW) programs, and an assistant professor at the University of Pennsylvania Perelman School of Medicine. She is a leading expert on improving population health through evidence-based CHW programs. Dr. Kangovi led the team that designed Individualized Management for Patient-Centered Targets (IMPaCT), a standardized, scalable CHW program, which has been delivered to nearly 10,000 high-risk patients and proven in three randomized controlled trials to improve chronic disease control, mental health, and quality of care while reducing total hospital days by 65 percent. The IMPaCT program has been disseminated to more than 1,000 organizations across the country and is being replicated by the Department of Veterans Affairs, state Medicaid programs, and large integrated health care organizations in rural and urban settings. Dr. Kangovi has authored numerous scientific publications, including in *The New England Journal of Medicine, JAMA,* and *Health Affairs,* and received more than $20 million in funding, including grants from the National Institutes of Health and the Patient-Centered Outcomes Research Institute.

Laura Rasar King, Ed.D., M.P.H., serves as the executive director of the Council on Education for Public Health (CEPH). Dr. King has more than 15 years of experience leading public health and higher education organizations in their quality assurance and improvement efforts. Her work and career have focused on bridging the gap between the needs of the public health workforce and academic public health. Working with faculty, practitioners, alumni, academic administrators, and employers in a multiyear process, CEPH developed outcomes-focused accreditation criteria for both the M.P.H. and Dr.P.H. programs. These criteria require specific foundational competencies of all graduate students for the first time since the inception of accreditation in public health. Under her leadership, the organization has more than doubled the number of accredited public health schools and programs, initiated accreditation of undergraduate public health programs, and extended its reach internationally.

Dr. King has been integral to advancing workforce development efforts in public health through her professional activities. As a member of the National Board of Public Health Examiners since 2013, she served on the Job Task Analysis steering committee, which completed the first-ever survey and analysis of the tasks in which public health practitioners in all settings are engaged on a day-to-day basis. She participates regularly on task forces and work groups led by the Association of Schools and Programs of Public Health, advising on issues such as articulation between undergraduate and graduate public health education and innovations in pedagogy. She offered her accreditation expertise and supported the development of the Public Health Accreditation Board, serving on its Workforce Think Tank (2011–2013) and Assessment Process Work Group (2008–2014). She was also a member of the Division Board for Professional Development of the National Commission for Health Education Credentialing (2004–2009) and the National Task Force for Accreditation in Health Education. In addition, she has held a variety of appointed and elected positions in the American Public Health Association (APHA), including as a member of the education board. She was the 2002 Judith R. Miller Award recipient for service to the Public Health Education and Health Promotion section and APHA in support of the practice and profession of health education.

Dr. King also serves in a variety of capacities in the higher education accreditation community. She is the immediate past chair of the Association of Specialized and Professional Accreditors (ASPA), where she is also the chair of the Education Policy Committee. In her role with ASPA, she testified before the Senate Committee on Health, Education, Labor & Pensions about professional education and specialized accreditation and is currently the primary negotiator for specialized accreditation in the Accreditation and Innovation Negotiated Rulemaking process as regulations are developed for the Higher Education Act. She regularly advocates for professional education and its connection to workforce needs, especially in the health professions, and the importance of quality assurance programs at a national level. Dr. King is a frequent speaker on higher education, accreditation, academic public health, and public health workforce issues. She has published several articles in public health journals, including *American Journal of Public Health*, *Health Education & Behavior*, *Health Promotion Practice*, and *Frontiers in Public Health*.

Dr. King earned an Ed.D. in organizational development from Northeastern University. Her dissertation work focused on the development and design of Dr.P.H. programs in schools of public health. She holds an M.P.H. in health promotion and disease prevention from The George Washington University Milken Institute School of Public Health and a B.A. in psychology from American University.

Sanne Magnan, M.D., Ph.D.,† is the co-chair of the National Academies of Sciences, Engineering, and Medicine's Roundtable on Population Health Improvement. She is the former president (2006–2007) and the chief executive officer (2011–2016) of the Institute for Clinical Systems Improvement. In 2007, she was appointed the commissioner of the Minnesota Department of Health by Governor Tim Pawlenty. She served from 2007 to 2010 and had significant responsibility for implementing Minnesota's 2008 health reform legislation, including the Statewide Health Improvement Program, standardized quality reporting, development of provider peer grouping, certification process for health care homes, and baskets of care. Dr. Magnan was a staff physician at the Tuberculosis Clinic at St. Paul–Ramsey County Department of Public Health (2002–2015). She was a member of the Population-based Payment Model Workgroup of the Healthcare Payment Learning and Action Network (2015–2016) and the Centers for Medicare & Medicaid Services' Multisector Collaboration Measure Development Technical Expert Panel (2016). She is on Epic's

Population Health Steering Board and the Healthy People 2030 Engagement Subcommittee. She served on the boards of MN Community Measurement and NorthPoint Health & Wellness Center, a federally qualified health center and part of Hennepin Health. Her previous experience also includes serving as the vice president and the medical director of consumer health at Blue Cross and Blue Shield of Minnesota. Currently, she is a senior fellow with HealthPartners Institute and an adjunct assistant professor of medicine at the University of Minnesota. Dr. Magnan holds an M.D. and a Ph.D. in medicinal chemistry from the University of Minnesota and is a board-certified internist.

Phyllis D. Meadows, Ph.D., R.N., M.S.N.,*† a senior fellow in the Health Program, engages in all levels of grant-making activity. Since joining The Kresge Foundation in 2009, she has advised the health team on the development of its overall strategic direction and provided leadership in the design and implementation of grant-making initiatives and projects. Dr. Meadows has coached team members and created linkages to national organizations and experts in the health field. In addition, she regularly reviews grant proposals, aids prospective grantees in preparing funding requests, and provides health-related expertise. "As a health professional, it is gratifying to see that Kresge recognizes the importance of public health and has made a major commitment to investing in the sector," Dr. Meadows says. "This is a fabulous opportunity for me to work on the ground floor with a major national foundation in shaping the direction and scope of its philanthropic funding for health." Dr. Meadows's 30-year career spans the nursing, public health, academic, and philanthropic sectors. She is the associate dean for practice at the University of Michigan School of Public Health and has lectured at the Wayne State University School of Nursing, Oakland University School of Nursing, and Marygrove College. From 2004 to 2009, Dr. Meadows served as the deputy director, the director, and the public health officer at the Detroit Department of Health and Wellness Promotion. In the early 1990s, she traveled abroad as a Kellogg International Leadership Fellow and subsequently joined the W.K. Kellogg Foundation as a program director. She also served as the director of nursing for the Medical Team–Michigan.

Dwyan Monroe, CHW, the program coordinator of community health worker (CHW) initiatives with the Institute for Public Health Innovation (IPHI), is part of a team that designs, plans, and delivers training and technical assistance for programs, institutions, and health systems incorporating CHWs and outreach initiatives in the District of Columbia, Maryland, and Virginia region. She also coaches and supports all IPHI

CHWs and manages CHW trainings through the IPHI Center for the Community Health Workforce. IPHI and Ms. Monroe are both widely recognized in the region and nationally for their expertise related to CHWs.

A former CHW and current CHW master trainer, Ms. Monroe has nearly 25 years of experience as an advocate for the profession. In 2006, she was appointed the director of the New Jersey Community Health Worker Institute, a statewide federally funded initiative of the New Jersey Area Health Education Centers. She worked as a research program coordinator in several clinical and community-based research programs at Johns Hopkins University from 1997 to 2003. Ms. Monroe is a graduate of Hampton University with a B.A. in psychology. She has completed numerous certificate programs in public health leadership, community and clinical health outreach, and community-based program development.

Jeremy Moseley, M.P.H.,[*] attended the University of North Carolina at Chapel Hill and East Carolina University, with foci in public health, policy, analysis, and management. He worked for the North Carolina Division of Public Health for 4 years, Duke University, and other health care organizations before coming to Wake Forest Baptist Medical Center in 2011. He is the director of community engagement in FaithHealth.

Karen Murphy, Ph.D., M.B.A.,[*†] is the executive vice president, the chief innovation officer, and the founding director of The Steele Institute for Health Innovation at Geisinger. Dr. Murphy has worked to improve and transform health care delivery throughout her career in both the public and private sectors. Before joining Geisinger, she served as Pennsylvania's secretary of health and addressed the most significant health issues facing the state, including the opioid epidemic. Earlier, Dr. Murphy was the director of the State Innovation Models Initiative at the Centers for Medicare & Medicaid Services (CMS), leading a $990 million CMS investment designed to accelerate health care innovation across the United States. She previously served as the president and the chief executive officer (CEO) of the Moses Taylor Health Care System in Scranton and as the founder and the CEO of Physicians Health Alliance, Inc., an integrated medical group practice within Moses Taylor.

Dr. Murphy earned her Ph.D. in business administration from the Temple University Fox School of Business. She holds an M.B.A. from Marywood University, a B.S. in liberal arts from the University of Scranton, and a diploma in nursing from the Scranton State Hospital School of Nursing. An author and national speaker on health policy and innovation, Dr. Murphy also serves as a clinical faculty member at the Geisinger Commonwealth School of Medicine.

Adriana Rodriguez Palacios, CHW, is originally from Mexico City. She arrived in Oregon in her middle school years and has remained there ever since. Her work with *Promotores de Salud de la Iglesia* (translated as Church Community Health Workers) began in 2006. That work motivated her to continue her education in public health and simultaneously continue to advocate for community health workers (CHWs) in the workforce. In 2012, she joined her colleagues in the creation of the Oregon Community Health Workers Association, and she continues to serve on its board and work with the community as a CHW.

Kalpana Ramiah, Dr.P.H., M.P.H., has a well-established career in public health and health services research that spans two decades. She has extensive experience conducting research and managing federally and privately funded technical assistance projects and research programs. She is highly skilled in patient and family engagement, population health, and measures and materials development.

Before joining Essential Hospitals Institute, Dr. Ramiah was a principal researcher at the American Institutes for Research and an assistant research professor at The George Washington University (GWU). She managed several major projects in patient engagement, health promotion and disease prevention, quality improvement, cost and coverage, and equity. At GWU, Dr. Ramiah oversaw the technical assistance portfolio of the Robert Wood Johnson Foundation's Aligning Forces for Quality.

Dr. Ramiah holds a Dr.P.H. and M.P.H. from GWU and bachelor's and master's degrees in nutrition. Dr. Ramiah is part of a number of national advisory committees and technical expert panels.

Michael Rhein, M.P.A., is the president and the chief executive officer of the Institute for Public Health Innovation (IPHI). As the official public health institute serving the District of Columbia, Maryland, and Virginia, IPHI develops multi-sector partnerships and innovative solutions to improve the public's health and well-being across the region, with a focus on strengthening health systems and policy, enhancing community conditions that promote health, and building community capacity to ensure equitable health opportunities for all. Mr. Rhein was involved in launching IPHI in 2009–2010 and has led its first decade of growth and success.

Mr. Rhein's public health career spans 25 years with such organizations as CommonHealth ACTION, the National AIDS Fund, the National Association of County and City Health Officials, and the Metropolitan Washington Council of Governments. His experience ranges from developing and implementing large-scale national initiatives to working alongside community organizations to design and implement effective public health efforts at a local level. Throughout his career, he has served in intermediary roles, helping to broker public and private resources and facilitate practical support for communities. This has involved collaborating with large national private foundations and corporations; federal, state, and local government agencies; local foundations; academia; health care providers; community-based organizations; and other partners across the country and locally in the District of Columbia, Maryland, and Virginia region.

Anna Ricklin, M.H.S., AICP, is a passionate advocate for healthy communities. She currently serves as the first health in all policies manager for the Fairfax County Health Department in Fairfax, Virginia, where she acts as a health ambassador across county agencies. In this role, Ms. Ricklin promotes the integration of public health objectives into county plans, policies, and building projects. Formerly, Ms. Ricklin led the American Planning Association Planning and Community Health Center, where she oversaw applied research and place-based initiatives to advance healthy planning practice. She has a background in health impact assessment, active transportation planning, and cross-sector collaboration, as well as recent work establishing metrics for healthy planning. Ms. Ricklin holds an M.H.S. from the Johns Hopkins Bloomberg School of Public Health and is based in Washington, DC.

Sagar Shah, Ph.D., AICP, is a research associate at the American Planning Association (APA) Planning and Community Health Center. He holds a doctorate in regional development planning from the University of Cincinnati with a focus on healthy urban planning. Dr. Shah is currently involved in applied research projects at APA, connecting urban planning and public health. Previously, he worked on the Centers for Disease Control and Prevention–funded Communities Putting Prevention to Work program, where he contributed his planning expertise and collaborated closely with the local health department and community partners. His research interest includes investigating the complex relationship between the built environment and health through a social equity lens.

Joshua M. Sharfstein, M.D.,*† is the vice dean for public health practice and community engagement and a professor of the practice in health policy and management at the Johns Hopkins Bloomberg School of Public Health. He is also the director of the Bloomberg American Health Initiative. His book, *Public Health Crisis Survival Guide: Leadership and Management in Trying Times*, was published by Oxford University Press in 2018. Previously, Dr. Sharfstein served as the secretary of the Maryland Department of Health and Mental Hygiene from January 2011 to December 2014.

In this position, he led efforts to align Maryland's health care system with improved health outcomes, culminating in the adoption of a revised payment model for all hospital care for Maryland residents. He also oversaw the development of a statewide health improvement process with 18 local public–private coalitions and the reshaping of the state's approach to health information exchange, long-term care, and behavioral health. From March 2009 to January 2011, Dr. Sharfstein was the principal deputy commissioner of the Food and Drug Administration, where he oversaw the agency's successful performance management and transparency initiatives. From December 2005 to March 2009, as the commissioner of health for Baltimore City, Dr. Sharfstein led innovative efforts that contributed to major declines in both overdose deaths and infant mortality rates. From July 2001 to December 2005, as the minority professional staff and health policy advisor for Congressman Henry A. Waxman, Dr. Sharfstein was engaged in a wide range of oversight and legislative activities on health care topics, including emergency preparedness, HIV, and the politicization of science.

Dr. Sharfstein graduated summa cum laude with an A.B. in social studies from Harvard College in 1991. From August 1991 to August 1992, he worked on public health projects in Guatemala and Costa Rica with a Frederick Sheldon Traveling Fellowship. He graduated from Harvard Medical School in 1996, from the Boston Combined Residency Program in Pediatrics at the Boston Medical Center and Children's Hospital in 1999, and from the fellowship in general academic pediatrics at the Boston University School of Medicine in 2001. Dr. Sharfstein is an elected fellow of the National Academy of Medicine (2014) and the National Academy of Public Administration (2013). He serves on the National Academies of Sciences, Engineering, and Medicine's Health and Medicine Division's Board of Population Health and Public Health Practice and the editorial board of *JAMA*. His awards have included the Jay S. Drotman Memorial Award from the American Public Health Association (1994), Public Official of the Year from *Governing Magazine* (2008), and the Circle of Commendation Award from the Consumer Product Safety Commission (2013).

Brian D. Smedley, Ph.D., is the co-founder and the executive director of the National Collaborative for Health Equity, a project that connects research, policy analysis, and communications with on-the-ground activism to advance health equity. In this role, Dr. Smedley oversees several initiatives designed to improve opportunities for good health for people of color and undo the health consequences of racism. From 2008 to 2014, Dr. Smedley was the vice president and the director of the Health Policy Institute of the Joint Center for Political and Economic Studies in Washington, DC, a research and policy organization focused on addressing the needs of communities of color.

Michelle Spencer, Ph.D., is the associate director of the Bloomberg American Health Initiative and an associate scientist within the Department of Health Policy and Management at the Johns Hopkins Bloomberg School of Public Health. She has more than 20 years of experience in public health management and leadership and a wealth of experience in administrative and operational management, strategic planning, resource management, and policy development. She previously served as the director of the Prevention and Health Promotion Administration at the Maryland Department of Health and Mental Hygiene and the director of the Maryland Health Enterprise Zone initiative. She oversaw the department's core public health programs, which included maternal and child health, infectious disease epidemiology and outbreak response, infectious disease prevention and health services, environmental health, and primary care and community health. Ms. Spencer focuses on addressing the preventable nature of public health issues through integrated, evidence-based approaches, with an emphasis on reducing disparities and advancing health equity. She was the chief of staff of the Baltimore Health Department from 2004–2012.

Noelle Wiggins, Ed.D., M.S., is the senior research and evaluation consultant for the Oregon Community Health Workers Association (ORCHWA) and a consultant in private practice. She has had the pleasure and honor of working with community health workers (CHWs) and *promotores/ promotoras* for more than 30 years. She began her work with CHWs in a rural area of El Salvador, where she lived from 1986 to 1990. From 1990 to 1995, Dr. Wiggins directed La Familia Sana ("The Healthy Family"), a CHW program in the migrant and seasonal working community in Hood River, Oregon. She served as the associate director of the landmark 1998 National Community Health Advisor Study and the lead author on the chapter on the roles and competencies of CHWs. Dr. Wiggins founded the Community Capacitation Center at the Multnomah County Health Department in Portland, Oregon, and directed that program for 18 years. She is a co-founder of ORCHWA and a past president of the Oregon Public Health Association. She has published multiple peer-reviewed articles and presented at many conferences.

She is passionate about using popular/people's education for CHW training, preparing CHWs to play a wide range of roles, supporting professional development for CHWs, and engaging CHWs in community-based participatory research and evaluation. Thanks to financial aid, Dr. Wiggins earned a B.A. in history with honors from Yale University, an

M.S. from the Harvard T.H. Chan School of Public Health, and an Ed.D. from Portland State University.

Katie Wunderlich, M.P.P., began her tenure as the executive director of the Health Services Cost Review Commission (HSCRC) in September 2018, where she led the commission through the transition from the hospital-based, all-payer model to the total cost of care model, which focuses on hospital and nonhospital system transformation that enhances patient care, improves health, and lowers costs. Previously, Ms. Wunderlich was the principal deputy director at HSCRC, overseeing the Center for Provider Alignment and Engagement, which works with hospitals, physicians, and other health care providers in partnership with patients to achieve the goals of the new model and transform health care delivery. She also directs legislative advocacy efforts for HSCRC for issues before the Maryland General Assembly and with Maryland's congressional delegation. Before joining HSCRC in 2016, Ms. Wunderlich was a deputy legislative officer in Governor Hogan's legislative office. She also served as the director of government relations for the Maryland Hospital Association and as a budget analyst for the General Assembly's Legislative Services Department. She holds an M.P.P. from The George Washington University.

Appendix D

Small Group Exercise Instructions and Worksheet

Tabletop Exercise: Toward a Population Health Workforce

Issue	Go with the issue group identified on your packet: 1. School absenteeism 2. Affordable housing 3. Food security	
Convener(s)	Who will be the convener? (e.g., county executive; regional health system; major regional nonprofit [e.g., Y organization or a chamber of commerce])	*Suggestions:* • Consider circumstances where an "honest broker" could be helpful. • Convener invites people to the table, with attention to power imbalances, and considers the levers each participant can activate.
Broad "approach"	The broad approach (e.g., multi-faceted solution to the issue) does not need to be specified but refers to the higher-order initiative or effort that workforce strategies are part of (e.g., a collective impact effort, a community development plan) **Strategies:** (e.g., a workforce plan, communication campaign, training program, [under]graduate dual degree program) **Tactics:** (e.g., CHW training, advocacy training, HIA training; public education effort or community deliberation; on-the-job certification [HIA, land use]; dual degree curriculum) **Responsible partner(s):** place of worship, school of public health, community-based organization, foundation, CDFI, supermarket, other business, health system	*Suggestions:* • Consider that for the three broad issues identified above, a workforce strategy will generally be part of a broader approach (e.g., a major initiative for policy change, economic development). • Set the context for the broader approach, but your focus should be on the workforce strategies that will be needed. Identify tactics and partners for each. • Try to include all three categories on today's agenda (e.g., health sector, CHWs and others, cross-sector) in your workforce strategies.

continued

Tabletop Exercise Continued

Funding	How will you pay for this? (e.g., community benefit, property tax, new market tax credit, government or foundation grant, financing package from public and private sources)

NOTE: CDFI = community development financial institution; CHW = community health worker; HIA = health impact assessment.

Given your background and what you heard today, how would you approach the issue? Draw on any knowledge you have of an evidence base that supports particular initiatives/approaches.

If you are a community health worker/educator/health official, you could play that role. Or, if a different role is needed in your group, draw on your knowledge to role-play that.

Please apply a health equity perspective to your discussion and role-play.

1 EDUCATION

Chronic absenteeism (missing 10 percent or more of school days[1] or 15 days or more)[2] is a major challenge in Ourtown, USA, population 250,000. About one in four children in Ourtown public schools miss 20.5 or more days of school per year. School absenteeism has been found to be four times higher in students from low-income families, where factors such as housing instability or inadequacy, health issues (e.g., asthma), safety concerns, and family unemployment can be important contributors. For children, absenteeism is associated with delayed reading, school failure, and dropout. Children who are absent in preschool, kindergarten, or first grade are much less likely to read at grade level by third grade and four times more likely to drop out of school. Absenteeism is associated with a loss of state funding for schools, which can amount to hundreds of thousands of dollars each year, limiting their ability to provide adequate educational resources to pupils.[3]

Last month, a summit on absenteeism was convened. The opening speaker asked "Whose primary job is it to focus on absenteeism?";

---

[1] See https://www2.ed.gov/datastory/chronicabsenteeism.html (accessed April 30, 2021).
[2] See https://healthyschoolscampaign.org/wp-content/uploads/2018/10/Education-Data-for-Health-Systems-Report-10-9-18.pdf (accessed April 30, 2021).
[3] See https://www.rwjf.org/en/library/research/2016/09/the-relationship-between-school-attendance-and-health.html (accessed April 30, 2021).

nobody raised a hand. Educators said their job was to teach students, clinicians said their job was to provide medical attention, and community leaders said their job was to support families through job training and other economic development.

Assembled leaders urged the county executive to call for a plan to end absenteeism. Under that plan, please describe workforce strategies and tactics and designate the partner(s) responsible for each. Then, explain how a newly empowered workforce across all three areas (if desired, or pick one) can come together and be held accountable in support of this effort. Please also add your suggestions for how this plan could be financed.

2 AFFORDABLE HOUSING

Housing affordability is a major concern in Ourtown, USA. Areas of this city of 500,000 are rapidly gentrifying, and high-priced condominiums are displacing lifelong residents. Rent prices have increased by more than 50 percent over the past 5 years, and incomes have not kept up for many city residents—nearly 60 percent of Ourtown residents are rent burdened, meaning that their rent consumes more than half of their income. Combined with a growing population of unhoused residents, the need for housing has never been greater.[4]

Over the past several years, local social services organizations, the health department, and the media have called attention to the growing housing crisis in the city. A wide range of partners came together to identify an approach to expand truly affordable housing in Ourtown. The facilitator at the kickoff meeting asked "Whose primary job is housing?" The department of housing and community development said "it's our main job, but we can't do it alone." The health system chief executive officer said that its community health needs assessment (and extensive news media coverage) had identified housing as a major need and also learned that 10 percent of emergency department admissions are either homeless or at risk of homelessness,[5] and after further research and dialogue, the system's board decided to make a major investment. "Housing clearly is a health issue," the hospital leadership said, "but we're not housing experts, and we're glad to be part of this broad coalition to tackle this issue." The area's renewable energy cooperative became involved with the emerging

---

[4] See https://www.fastcompany.com/90291860/this-healthcare-giant-invests-millions-in-affordable-housing-to-keep-people-healthy and https://www.mercurynews.com/2017/10/05/lifestyle-switch-more-bay-area-residents-are-choosing-to-rent-than-ever-before-and-theyre-paying-through-the-nose (accessed April 30, 2021).

[5] See https://www.ncbi.nlm.nih.gov/pmc/articles/PMC5391885 (accessed April 30, 2021).

housing coalition to inform efforts to make affordable housing sustainable for residents.

The coalition steering group called for a comprehensive affordable housing plan. Please describe workforce strategies and tactics and designate the partner(s) responsible for each. Then, explain how a newly empowered workforce across all three areas (if desired, or pick one) can come together to support and be held accountable for an expansion in affordable housing. Please also add your suggestions for how this plan could be financed.

3 FOOD SECURITY/HEALTHY FOOD

Food security is a health issue in Ourtown, USA, population 750,000. About one in five children live in a household that has difficulty getting enough food and especially with obtaining fresh produce. The city has also lost a grocery store, which has left one area without reliable access to fresh food options. Associated with this challenge, city residents experience an obesity rate higher than in the average American city.

The major local community nonprofit convened a group of stakeholders and partners to discuss the issue and consider the options for strengthening the local food environment to tackle both food insecurity and poor health outcomes associated with obesity. For example, the local school district has not adopted the community eligibility provision of Title I (of the Every Student Succeeds Act), which would reduce the administrative burden on schools with low-income students who would benefit from free and reduced-price breakfast and lunch. To implement a healthy food environment strategy, the partners assembled identified some areas where communication, orientation, and training could equip all types of workers with knowledge and skills to advocate and take action in ways that can help address this community need.

The group called for a comprehensive food security/healthy food plan. Please describe workforce strategies and tactics and designate the partner(s) responsible for each. Then, explain how a newly empowered workforce across all three areas (if desired, or pick one) can come together and be held accountable in support of this effort. Please also add your suggestions for how this plan could be financed.

APPENDIX D

Fill in the table based on your discussion, and choose someone to report back.

Small group worksheet (to be completed by scribe and read by the facilitator/rapporteur)

Issue:		
Convener(s):		
Partners:		
Approach: (may leave blank)		
Strategies	Tactics	Responsible Partner
1.		
2.		
3.		
4.		